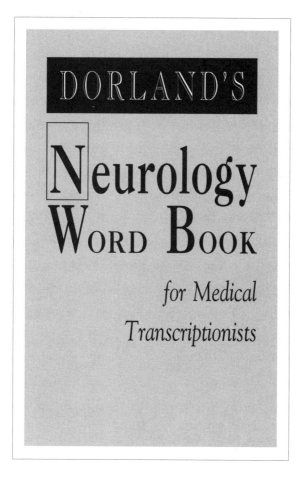

DORLAND'S

Neurology
WORD BOOK

for Medical

Transcriptionists

DORLAND'S

Neurology WORD BOOK

for Medical Transcriptionists

Series Editor
SHARON B. RHODES, CMT, RHIT

Edited & Reviewed by:
Ann Marie Donnelly, CMT, MS

W.B. SAUNDERS COMPANY
A Harcourt Health Sciences Company

Philadelphia   London   New York   St. Louis   Sydney   Toronto

W.B. Saunders Company
A Harcourt Health Sciences Company

The Curtis Center
Independence Square West
Philadelphia, Pennsylvania 19106

Dorland's Neurology Word Book for
Medical Transcriptionists

ISBN 0-7216-9078-5

Printed in the United States of America.

Last digit is the print number: 9 8 7 6 5 4 3 2 1

I am proud to present the *Dorland's Neurology Word Book for Medical Transcriptionists*—part of a series of word books compiled for the professional medical transcriptionist. For one hundred years, W.B. Saunders has published the *Dorland's Illustrated Medical Dictionary.* With the advent of medical transcription, it became the dictionary of choice for medical transcriptionists.

When approached last year to help develop a new series of word books for W.B. Saunders, I have to admit the thought absolutely overwhelmed me. The *Dorland's Illustrated Medical Dictionary* was one of my first book purchases when I began my transcription career over thirty years ago. To be invited to participate in this project is an honor I could never have imagined for myself!

Transcriptionists need and will continue to need trusted up-to-date resources to help them research difficult terms quickly. In developing the *Dorland's Neurology Word Book for Medical Transcriptionists,* I had access to the entire *Dorland's* terminology database for the book's foundation. In addition to this immense database, a context editor, Ann Donnelly, CMT, MS, a H.O.P.E. mentor for the Epilepsy Foundation and a recognized expert in the field of neurology transcription, was selected to review the material from the database, to contribute new and unique terms, and to remove outdated and obsolete ones. With Ann's extensive research and diligent work, I believe this to be the most up-to-date word book for the field of neurology.

In developing the neurology word book, I wanted the size to be manageable so the book would be easy to handle, with a durable, long-lasting binding, and using a type font large enough to read while providing extensive terminology. Anatomical plates displaying neuroanatomy of the brain and nervous system were also added.

Although I have tried to produce the most thorough word book for neurology available to medical transcriptionists, it is difficult to include every term as the field of neurology is constantly evolving. As you discover new terms, please feel free to share them with me for inclusion in the next edition of the *Dorland's Neurology Word Book for Medical Transcriptionists.*

I may be reached at the following e-mail address: Sharon@TheRhodes.com.

SHARON B. RHODES, CMT, RHIT
Brentwood, Tennessee

A
 A delta fibers
 A fibers
 A wave

AI area

AII area

Abadie's sign

abaptiston

abarognosis

abasia
 a. atactica
 ataxic a.
 choreic a.
 paralytic a.
 paroxysmal trepidant a.
 spastic a.
 trembling a.
 a. trepidans

abasic

abatic

abdomen
 boat-shaped a.
 carinate a.
 navicular a.
 scaphoid a.

abducens

abducent

abduct

abduction

abductor

aberrant

abetalipoproteinemia

abirritation

abmortal

aboulia

Abrams' heart reflex

abscess
 brain a.

abscess *(continued)*
 epidural a.
 extradural a.
 frontal a.
 intradural a.
 subdural a.

absence

abulia

acalculia

acanthesthesia

acaudal

acaudate

accelerator

accident
 cerebrovascular a.

accommodation
 nerve a.

acedia

acephaly

acetaminophen

acetylcholine

acheiria, achiria

Achilles
 A. jerk
 A. tendon reflex
 A. tendon reflex time

achondroplasia

achromia
 cortical a.

acinesia

acinetic

acoasma

acoria

acousma

acousmatamnesia

acoustic

acousticophobia

acroagnosis

acroanesthesia

acroasphyxia

acroataxia

acroesthesia

acrognosis

acroneurosis

acroparalysis

acroparesthesia

acropathy
    ulcerative mutilating a.

acrotrophodynia

acrotrophoneurosis

act
    reflex a.

ACTH
    adrenocorticotropic hor-
        mone
            ACTH-producing ade-
                noma

action
    a. potential
    reflex a.

activation
    a. procedure

activity
    alpha a.
    background a.
    beta a.
    continuous muscle a.
    continuous muscle fiber a.
    a's of daily living (ADL)
    delta a.
    electrical a.
    end-plate a.
    epileptiform a.
    insertion a.
    insertional a.

activity *(continued)*
    intermittent rhythmic del-
        ta a.
    polymorphic delta a.
    salaam a.
    spontaneous a.
    transient a.
    theta a.

adamantinoma
    pituitary a.

adaptation

Adderall

Addison's disease

adendric

adendritic

adenoma *pl.* adenomas, adeno-
    mata
    ACTH-producing a.
    chromophobe a.
    growth hormone–produ-
        cing a.

adenoneural

adenopituicyte

adhesio *pl.* adhesiones
    a. interthalamica

adhesion
    interthalamic a.

adiadochocinesia

adiadochocinesis

adiadochokinesia

adiadochokinesis

adiadokokinesia

adiadokokinesis

adiaphoria

Adie
    A's pupil
    A's syndrome

adiposis
    a. cerebralis

adiposity
    cerebral a.
    pituitary a.

adipsia

ADL
    activities of daily living

admixed

adnerval

adneural

adrenaline

adrenergic

adrenoceptive

adrenoceptor

adrenoleukodystrophy

adrenolytic

adrenomimetic

adrenoreceptor

adromia

Adson
    A's maneuver
    A's test

adynamia

adynamic

AED
    antiepileptic drug

aerocele
    epidural a.
    intracranial a.

aesthetic

affect
    blunted a.
    constricted a.
    flat a.
    inappropriate a.
    labile a.
    restricted a.

affective
    a. disorder

afferent
    a. sensory

afterbrain

afterdepolarization
    delayed a.
    early a.
    late a.

afterdischarge

afterimpression

afterperception

afterpotential
    negative a.
    positive a.

aftersensation

aftertaste

aftertouch

aganglionic

age
    a.-associated memory impairment
    a.-related memory impairment
    developmental a.
    mental a.

agenesia
    a. corticalis

agenesis
    corpus callosum a.
    nuclear a.

ageusia

ageusic

ageustia

agitographia

agitophasia

aglomerular

agnea

agnosia
    acoustic a.

agnosia *(continued)*
    auditory a.
    body-image a.
    face a.
    facial a.
    finger a.
    ideational a.
    posture a.
    tactile a.
    time a.
    visual a.

agonist

agouti

agrammatica

agrammatism

agrammatologia

agraphia
    absolute a.
    acoustic a.
    alexia without a.
    a. amnemonica
    a. atactica
    cerebral a.
    jargon a.
    literal a.
    mental a.
    motor a.
    musical a.
    optic a.
    verbal a.

agraphic

agyria

agyric

Aicardi
    A's syndrome
    A.-Goutieres syndrome

AIDS
    acquired immunodeficiency
      syndrome
        AIDS dementia com-
          plex
        AIDS encephalopathy

akathisia

akinesia

akinesis

akinesthesia

akinetic
    a. mutism

akoria

Akureyri disease

ala *pl.* alae
    a. of central lobule
    a. cerebelli
    alae lingulae cerebelli
    a. lobuli centralis

Alagille syndrome

Albright syndrome

Alexander's disease

alexia
    a. without agraphia
    cortical a.
    motor a.
    musical a.
    optical a.
    subcortical a.

alexic

algesia

algesic

algesichronometer

algesimeter
    Björnström's a.
    Boas' a.

algesimetry

algesiogenic

algesiometer

algesthesia

algesthesis

algetic

algiomotor

algiomuscular

algodystrophy

algogenesia

algogenesis

algogenic

algometer
    pressure a.

algometry

allachesthesia

allantoidean

allantois

Allen
    A's maneuver
    A's rule

allesthesia

allocheiria

allochesthesia

allochiral

allochiria

allocortex

allodynia

alloesthesia

allokinesis

allokinetic

all or none

allotriogeustia

allotriosmia

Alpers' disease

Alport's syndrome

alveus *pl.* alveus
    a. hippocampi
    a. of hippocampus

Alzheimer
    A's cells
    A's dementia
    dementia of the A. type

Alzheimer *(continued)*
    A's disease
    A's neurofibrillary degener-
    ation

amantadine

amaurosis
    cat's eye a.
    central a.
    a. centralis
    cerebral a.
    a. fugax

amaurotic

ambidexterity

ambidextrism

ambidextrous

ambilevosity

ambilevous

ambisinister

ambisinistrous

amblyaphia

amblygeustia

amblyope

amblyopia

ameloblastoma
    pituitary a.

amentia

Amerge

amiculum *pl.* amicula
    a. olivare
    a. of olive

amimia

amine
    biogenic a.

aminergic

amino acid
    excitatory a. a's

γ-aminobutyric acid

amitriptyline

Ammon
   horn of A.

ammonotelic

amnesia
   neurological a.
   postconcussional a.
   post-traumatic a.
   tactile a.
   transient global a.
   traumatic a.
   visual a.

amniote

amorphosynthesis

amphibious

amphicyte

amphotony

amusia
   instrumental a.
   sensory a.
   vocal motor a.

amyelinic

amygdala

amygdalohippocampectomy

amyloid
   a. neuropathy
   a. polyneuropathy

amyloidosis
   familial a.
   hereditary a.
   hereditary neuropathic a.
   heredofamilial a.

amyoesthesia

amyoesthesis

amyostasia

amyostatic

amyotonia

anacatesthesia

analgesia
   a. algera
   paretic a.

analgesic
   a. rebound headache

analgetic

analgia

analgic

analyzer

anamniote

anamniotic

anaphia

Anaprox

anaptic

anarithmia

anarthria

anastomosis
   Galen's a.
   Hyrtl's a.

Andermann syndrome

Andersch
   A's ganglion
   A's nerve

Andersen's syndrome

Anderson's disease

Andrade
   A's syndrome
   A. type familial amyloid
      polyneuropathy

André Thomas sign

anelectrotonic

anelectrotonus

anencephaly

anesthecinesia

anesthekinesia

anesthesia
    angiospastic a.
    bulbar a.
    compression a.
    crossed a.
    dissociated a.
    dissociation a.
    a. dolorosa
    facial a.
    gauntlet a.
    girdle a.
    glove a.
    gustatory a.
    muscular a.
    nausea a.
    olfactory a.
    peripheral a.
    pressure a.
    segmental a.
    spinal a.
    tactile a.
    thalamic hyperesthetic a.
    thermal a.
    traumatic a.
    unilateral a.
    visceral a.

anesthetic

aneurogenic

aneurysm
    berry a.
    brain a.
    cerebral a.
    congenital cerebral a.
    intracranial a.
    suprasellar a.

Angelman's syndrome

angiitis
    granulomatous a. of central
      nervous system
    isolated a. of central ner-
      vous system

angioblastoma

angioma *pl.* angiomas, angio-
  mata
    arteriovenous a. of brain

angioma *(continued)*
    cavernous a.
    venous a. of brain

angiomatosis
    cerebroretinal a.
    encephalofacial a.
    encephalotrigeminal a.
    retinocerebral a.

angioneuropathic

angioneuropathy

angioneurotic

angioparalysis

angioparesis

angiopathy
    cerebral amyloid a.
    congophilic a.

angiophakomatosis

angioreticuloma

angle
    cephalic-medullary a.
    cerebellopontine a.
    rolandic a.
    a. of Rolando
    sphenoid a.
    sphenoidal a.
    tentorial a.
    a. of Sylvius

anhaphia

anile

anility

animal
    decerebrate a.
    hyperphagic a.
    spinal a.
    thalamic a.

anisodont

annulus *pl.* annuli
    Vieussens' a.

anodmia

anomaly
    Aristotle's a.

anomia

anorthography

anosmatic

anosmia
    a. gustatoria
    preferential a.

anosmic

anosognosia

anosphresia

ansa *pl.* ansae
    a. cervicalis
    a. lenticularis
    ansae nervorum spinalium
    a. peduncularis
    a. subclavia
    a. of Vieussens

antagonist
    a. medication

anthrax
    cerebral a.
    meningeal a.

antiadrenergic

antibody
    anti-Hu a.
    anti-Ri a.
    anti-Yo a.

anticholinergic

anticonvulsant

antidromic

antiepileptic
    a. drug (AED)

antinociceptive

antiparasympathomimetic

antisympathetic

antitrismus

Antivert

Antley-Bixler syndrome

Anton
    A's symptom
    A's syndrome
    A.-Babinski syndrome

anuran

anurous

apallesthesia

aparalytic

Apert syndrome

apertura *pl.* aperturae
    a. lateralis ventriculi quarti
    a. mediana ventriculi quarti

aperture
    lateral a. of fourth ventricle
    median a. of fourth ventricle
    superior and inferior a's of axillary fossa

apex *pl.* apices
    a. cornus dorsalis medullae spinalis
    a. cornus posterioris medullae spinalis
    a. of dorsal horn of spinal cord
    a. of posterior horn of spinal cord

aphasia
    acoustic a.
    acquired epileptic a.
    amnesic a.
    amnestic a.
    anomic a.
    associative a.
    auditory a.
    Broca's a.
    central a.
    combined a.
    commissural a.
    complete a.
    conduction a.
    expressive a.

aphasia *(continued)*
    expressive-receptive a.
    fluent a.
    frontocortical a.
    gibberish a.
    global a.
    graphomotor a.
    impressive a.
    intellectual a.
    jargon a.
    mixed a.
    motor a.
    nominal a.
    nonfluent a.
    receptive a.
    semantic a.
    sensory a.
    syntactical a.
    tactile a.
    total a.
    transcortical a.
    true a.
    visual a.
    Wernicke's a.

aphasiac

aphasic

aphasiology

aphemesthesia

aphemia

aphonia

aphonogelia

aphose

aphrasia

aplacental

aplasia
    nuclear a.

apnea
    sleep a.
    sleep a., central
    sleep a., obstructive

apneusis

apneustic

apophysis
    cerebral a.
    a. cerebri

apoplectic

apoplectiform

apoplectoid

apoplexia

apoplexy
    bulbar a.
    cerebellar a.
    cerebral a.
    embolic a.
    pituitary a.
    pontile a.
    pontine a.
    Raymond's a.
    spinal a.
    thrombotic a.

apparatus
    Brown-Roberts-Wells a.
    Leksell a.
    a. of Perroncito
    Riechert-Mundinger a.
    subneural a.
    sucker a.
    Todd-Wells a.

appestat

apractagnosia

apractic

apraxia
    akinetic a.
    amnestic a.
    Bruns' a. of gait
    buccofacial a.
    classic a.
    Cogan's oculomotor a.
    congenital oculomotor a.
    constructional a.
    dressing a.
    facial a.
    ideational a.
    ideokinetic a.

apraxia *(continued)*
    ideomotor a.
    innervatory a.
    Liepmann's a.
    motor a.
    oculomotor a.
    sensory a.
    a. of speech
    transcortical a.

apraxic

apyknomorphous

aqueduct
    cerebral a.
    a. of mesencephalon
    a. of midbrain
    a. of Sylvius
    ventricular a.

aqueductus
    a. cerebri
    a. mesencephali

arachnitis

arachnoid
    a. of brain
    cranial a.
    spinal a.
    a. of spinal cord

arachnoidal

arachnoidea
    a. encephali
    a. spinalis

arachnoidea mater
    a. m. cranialis
    a. m. encephali
    a. m. spinalis
    a. m. et pia mater

arachnoiditis
    chronic adhesive a.
    neoplastic a.
    spinal a.

arachnoid mater
    cranial a. m.
    spinal a. m.

Aran
    A.-Duchenne disease
    A.-Duchenne muscular atrophy

Arantius
    ventricle of A.

arbor
    dendritic a.
    a. vitae
    a. vitae cerebelli

arborization

arc
    neural a.
    reflex a.
    sensorimotor a.

archaeocerebellum

archaeocortex

archeocerebellum

archeocortex

archicerebellum

archicortex

archipallial

archipallium

arc-quadrant

arcus
    a. parieto-occipitalis

area
    acoustic a's
    a. acustica
    AI a.
    AII a.
    a. amygdaloidea anterior
    anterior amygdaloid a.
    association a's
    auditory a's
    auditory association a.
    auditory receiving a's
    Betz cell a.
    brain a.
    Broca's motor speech a.

area *(continued)*
  Broca's parolfactory a.
  Brodmann's a's
  a. cerebrovasculosa
  cingulate a.
  cortical a.
  dermatomic a.
  entorhinal a.
  eye a.
  a. of facial nerve
  a's of Forel
  gustatory receiving a.
  hypothalamic a., anterior
  hypothalamic a., dorsal
  hypothalamic a., intermediate
  hypothalamic a., lateral
  hypothalamic a., posterior
  a. hypothalamica dorsalis
  a. hypothalamica intermedia
  a. hypothalamica lateralis
  a. hypothalamica posterior
  a. hypothalamica rostralis
  insular a.
  language a.
  a. medullovasculosa
  motor a.
  motor speech a.
  a. nervi facialis
  olfactory a.
  parastriate a.
  periamygdaloid a.
  peristriate a.
  piriform a.
  postcentral a.
  a. postrema
  postrolandic a.
  precentral a.
  prefrontal a.
  premotor a.
  preoptic a.
  a. preoptica
  prepiriform a.
  pretectal a.
  a. pretectalis
  primary a's
  primary motor a.
  primary receiving a's

area *(continued)*
  primary receptive a's
  primary somatomotor a.
  projection a's
  pyriform a.
  receptive a's
  a. retroolivaris
  retroolivary a.
  rolandic a.
  sensorimotor a.
  sensory a's.
  sensory association a.
  septal a.
  SI a.
  SII a.
  silent a.
  somatic sensory a.
  somatosensory a.
  somatosensory a., first
  somatosensory a., primary
  somatosensory a., second
  somatosensory a., secondary
  somesthetic a.
  striate a.
  strip a.
  a. subcallosa
  subcallosal a.
  supplementary a's
  supplementary motor a.
  suppressor a's
  taste receiving a.
  trigger a.
  vagus a.
  vestibular a.
  visual a.
  visual a., first
  visual a., second
  visual a., third
  visual association a's
  visual receiving a.
  visuopsychic a's
  visuosensory a.
  watershed a.
  Wernicke's a.
  Wernicke's second motor speech a.
areflexia

Aricept

Aristotle's anomaly

Armstrong's disease

Arnold
    A's canal
    A's nerve
    A's nerve reflex cough syn-
      drome
    A.-Chiari deformity
    A.-Chiari malformation
    A.-Chiari syndrome

arousal

arrhigosis

arrhythmokinesis

Artane

arterenol

arteriosclerosis
    cerebral a.

arteriovenous
    a. malformation (AVM)

arteritis *pl.* arteritides

artery
    posterior spinal a's
    posterior inferior a's

arthresthesia

arthritis *pl.* arthritides
    neuropathic a.

arthropathy
    Charcot's a.
    neurogenic a.
    neuropathic a.
    tabetic a.

artiodactylous

arylsulfatase A deficiency

asemasia

asemia

asomatognosia

aspartate

aspartic acid

assessment
    Fugl-Meyer a.

association

astasia

astatic

astereocognosy

astereognosis

asterixis

asthenia
    myalgic a.

asthenopia
    nervous a.

astroblast

astroblastoma

astrocyte
    fibrillary a's
    fibrous a's
    gemistocytic a.
    plasmatofibrous a's
    protoplasmic a's

astrocytoma
    anaplastic a.
    cerebellar a.
    diffuse cerebellar a.
    a. fibrillare
    fibrillary a.
    gemistocytic a.
    Grade I a's
    Grade II a's
    Grade III a's
    Grade IV a's
    juvenile pilocytic a.
    malignant a.
    pilocytic a.
    piloid a.
    protoplasmic a.
    a. protoplasmaticum
    subependymal giant cell a.

astrocytosis

astroglia

asyllabia

asymbolia
    pain a.

asymboly

asymmetry
    encephalic a.

asynchronism

asynchrony

asynergia

asynergic

asynergy

atactic

atactiform

ataxia
    acute a.
    acute cerebellar a.
    Bruns' frontal a.
    cerebellar a.
    cerebral a.
    childhood a. with cerebral
      hypomyelination
    Ferguson-Critchley a.
    Friedreich's a.
    frontal a.
    hereditary a.
    intrapsychic a.
    kinetic a.
    locomotor a.
    Menzel's a.
    motor a.
    Sanger Brown a.
    sensory a.
    spinal a.
    spinocerebellar a.
    a.-telangiectasia
    truncal a.

ataxiagram

ataxiagraph

ataxiameter

ataxiaphasia

ataxic

ataxy

athetoid

athetosic

athetosis
    double a.
    double congenital a.

athetotic

Ativan

atlas
    stereotactic a.

atonia
    choreatic a.

atonic
    a. seizure

atonicity

atony

atopognosia

atopognosis

atrophia
    a. musculorum lipomatosa

atrophy
    Aran-Duchenne muscular a.
    Charcot-Marie a.
    Charcot-Marie-Tooth a.
    circumscribed cerebral a.
    corticostriatospinal a.
    Cruveilhier's a.
    Dejerine-Sottas a.
    Dejerine-Thomas a.
    denervated muscle a.
    dentatorubral a.
    Duchenne-Aran muscular a.
    Eichhorst's a.
    Erb's a.
    facioscapulohumeral mus-
      cular a.
    Fazio-Londe a.
    Hoffmann's a.
    Hunt's a.

atrophy *(continued)*
    idiopathic muscular a.
    juvenile muscular a.
    Landouzy-Dejerine a.
    lobar a.
    multiple system a.
    myelopathic muscular a.
    neural a.
    neural muscular a.
    neuritic muscular a.
    neuropathic a.
    neurotrophic a.
    olivopontocerebellar a.
    pallidal a.
    peroneal a.
    peroneal muscular a.
    progressive muscular a.
    progressive neural muscular a.
    progressive neuromuscular a.
    pseudohypertrophic muscular a.
    segmental sensory dissociation with brachial muscular a.
    spinal muscular a.
    spinal muscular a., infantile
    spinal muscular a., juvenile
    spinal muscular a., progressive
    spinal muscular a., proximal
    spinal muscular a., Werdnig-Hoffmann
    Tooth's a.
    trophoneurotic a.
    Vulpian's a.
    white a.
    Zimmerlin's a.
attack
    drop a.
    panic a.
    transient ischemic a. (TIA)
    vagal a.
    vasovagal a.
atypical absence seizure

audition
    gustatory a.
auditory
    a. arteriovenous malformation
    a. AVM
    a. evoked potential
    a. seizure
    a. visual-evoked responses
    brain stem a. evoked potential
Auerbach's ganglion
aura
    auditory a.
    electric a.
    epigastric a.
    epileptic a.
    a. hysterica
    intellectual a.
    kinesthetic a.
    migraine a.
    migraine a. without headache
    motor a.
    reminiscent a.
    vertiginous a.
aural
auriculotherapy
Australian
    A. X disease
    A. X encephalitis
autoecholalia
automaticity
automatism
    spinal a's
automatograph
autonomic
autonomotropic
autosomal recessive syndrome of progressive encephalopathy

autosomatognosis

autosomatognostic

autotopagnosia

autotrepanation

Avellis
 A's paralysis
 A's syndrome

avifauna

AVM
 arteriovenous malforma-
  tion
   auditory AVM

Avonex

avulsion
 nerve a.

axifugal

axilemma

axipetal

axoaxonic

axodendritic

axofugal

axolemma

axolotl

axolysis

axon
 fusimotor a's
 giant a.
 myelinated a.
 naked a.
 unmyelinated a.

axonal

axonapraxia

axone

axonopathy
 distal a.
 proximal a.

axonotmesis

axopetal

axophage

axoplasm

axoplasmic

axosomatic

axotomy

Ayer
 A's test
 A.-Tobey test

Azorean disease

B
    B fibers

Babès
    B's nodes
    B's nodules
    B's tubercles

Babinski
    B's phenomenon
    B's reflex
    B's sign
    B's test
    B's toe sign
    B.-Nageotte syndrome

baclofen

baculum

bag
    nuclear b.

Baillarger
    external band of B.
    external line of B.
    inner band of B.
    inner line of B.
    internal band of B.
    internal line of B.
    outer band of B.
    outer line of B.
    B's sign

balance

Balint's syndrome

ball
    Marchi b's

Baller-Gerold syndrome

ballism

ballismus

ballistic

Baló's disease

Baltic myoclonus

16

Bamberger
    B's disease
    B's sign

band
    Baillarger's external b.
    Baillarger's inner b.
    Baillarger's internal b.
    Baillarger's outer b.
    b. of Broca
    Broca's diagonal b.
    Büngner's b's
    dentate b.
    diagonal b.
    diagonal b. of Broca
    external b. of Baillarger
    furrowed b.
    b. of Gennari
    Giacomini's b.
    inner b. of Baillarger
    internal b. of Baillarger
    oligoclonal b's
    outer b. of Baillarger
    Vicq d'Azyr's b.

bandaletta
    b. diagonalis (Broca)

Bannayan syndrome

Bannwarth's syndrome

baragnosis

Bárány
    B's maneuver
    B's pointing test

barba amarilla

Bardet-Biedl syndrome

baresthesia

baresthesiometer

Barker's point

Barkman's reflex

baroagnosis

baroceptor

barognosis

baroreceptor

Barré
- B's pyramidal sign
- B's sign
- B.-Guillain syndrome

barrier
- blood-brain b.
- blood-cerebral b.
- blood–cerebrospinal fluid b.
- hematoencephalic b.

Bartelmez
- club ending of B.

Barth syndrome

Bartter syndrome

baryesthesia

base
- b. of brain
- b. of dorsal horn of spinal cord
- b. of posterior horn of spinal cord

basis
- b. cerebri
- b. cornus dorsalis medullae spinalis
- b. cornus posterioris medullae spinalis
- b. pedunculi cerebri

Bassen-Kornzweig syndrome

Bastian
- B's law
- B.-Bruns law
- B.-Bruns sign

bat
- vampire b.

bathesthesia

bathmotropic
- negatively b.
- positively b.

bathmotropism

bathyanesthesia

bathyesthesia

bathyhyperesthesia

bathyhypesthesia

Batten disease

Battle's sign

Bayle's disease

Bechterev (see *Bekhterev*)

Becker
- B's disease
- B's muscular dystrophy
- B. type muscular dystrophy

Beckwith-Wiedemann syndrome

bed
- CircOlectric b.

Beevor's sign

Behçet disease

Behr syndrome

Bekhterev (Bekhterew)
- B's deep reflex
- B's layer
- B's nucleus
- B's reaction
- B's reflex
- B's sign
- B's test
- B's tract
- B-Mendel reflex

Bell
- B's nerve
- B's palsy
- B's paralysis
- B's phenomenon
- B's sign
- B's spasm

Bellergal

beneceptor

Benedikt's syndrome

benzodiazepine

Berardinelli syndrome

Bereitschaftspotential

Berger
   B. rhythm
   B's sign

Bergmann
   B's cells
   B's cords
   B's fibers
   B's glia
   B's rule

Bernard
   B's syndrome
   B.-Horner syndrome

Bernhardt
   B's disease
   B's paresthesia
   B.-Roth disease

beta
   b. blocker
   b. receptors

Betaseron

Betz
   B's cells
   B. cell area

bicoronal

Bidder
   B's ganglia
   B's organ

bidentate

Bielschowsky disease

Biernacki's sign

bigemina

bigeminum

bilirachia

Billroth's disease

bilophodont

bind
   double b.

Bing-Neel syndrome

Binswanger
   B's dementia
   B's disease
   B's encephalitis

bioamine

bioaminergic

bioelectricity

biohydraulic

biomechanics

bionics

biophysical

biophysics

biopsy
   stereotactic b.

biopsychology

biothesiometer

bipolar

birefringence
   crystalline b.
   flow b.
   form b.
   intrinsic b.
   strain b.
   streaming b.

birefringent

Bischof's myelotomy

Björnström's algesimeter

blackout

bladder
   allantoic b.
   neurogenic b.

Blake's pouch

Blandin's ganglion

blindness
: amnesic color b.
: cortical b.
: letter b.
: music b.
: object b.
: psychic b.
: taste b.
: text b.
: word b.

Bloch-Sulzberger syndrome

block
: anodal b.
: conduction b.
: depolarization b.
: dynamic b.
: motor point b.
: nerve b.
: neurolytic b.
: phenol b.
: phenol motor point b.
: spinal b.
: spinal subarachnoid b.
: ventricular b.

blockade
: neuromuscular b.

blocker
: beta b.

Blocq's disease

blood
: b.-brain barrier
: b.-cerebral barrier
: b.–cerebrospinal fluid barrier

Bloom syndrome

blue
: Luxol fast b. MBS
: solvent b. 38

Blumenau's nucleus

Boas' algesimeter

Bochdalek
: B's ganglion

Bochdalek *(continued)*
: B's pseudoganglion

Bock
: B's ganglion
: B's nerve

body
: amygdaloid b.
: b. of caudate nucleus
: b. of cerebellum
: chromophilous b's
: b. of fornix
: geniculate b., lateral
: geniculate b., medial
: habenular b.
: Harting b's
: Herring b's
: Hirano b's
: infundibular b.
: interrenal b.
: juxtarestiform b.
: Lafora's b's
: b. of lateral ventricle
: Lewy b's
: Luys' b.
: mammillary b.
: mammillary b.
: medullary b. of cerebellum
: medullary b. of vermis
: Nissl b's
: olivary b.
: pacchionian b's
: paraterminal b.
: parietal b.
: parolivary b's
: Pick b's
: pineal b.
: pineal b.
: pituitary b.
: quadrigeminal b's
: Reilly b's
: Renaut's b's
: restiform b.
: sand b's
: striate b.
: tigroid b's
: Todd b's
: trapezoid b.

body *(continued)*
  Verocay b's
  zebra b.

Boehme disease

Bonhoeffer's symptom

Bonnet
  B's sign
  B.-Dechaum-Blanc syn-
    drome

Bordier-Fränkel sign

Bouchet-Gsell disease

bouffée délirante

bouton
  b. de passage
  b. en passant
  synaptic b.
  b. terminal

Bowditch's law

bracelet
  Nageotte's b's

brachialgia
  b. statica paresthetica

brachium *pl.* brachia
  b. of caudal colliculus
  b. colliculi caudalis
  b. colliculi inferioris
  b. colliculi rostralis
  b. colliculi superioris
  b. of inferior colliculus
  b. opticum
  b. pontis
  b. of rostral colliculus
  b. of superior colliculus

brachybasia

bradyarthria

bradycinesia

bradyesthesia

bradyglossia

bradykinesia

bradylalia

bradylexia

bradylogia

bradyphasia

bradyphrasia

bradyphrenia

bradypragia

bradyteleocinesia

bradyteleokinesis

Bragard's sign

Brain's reflex

brain
  olfactory b.
  respirator b.
  split b.
  smell b.
  wet b.

brainstem

branch
  anterior b. of axillary nerve
  anterior b's of thoracic
    nerves
  articular b. of deep fibular
    nerve
  circumferential b's
  communicating b. with cili-
    ary ganglion
  communicating b. with na-
    sociliary nerve
  communicating b. of naso-
    ciliary nerve with ciliary
    ganglion
  b. to coracobrachialis
  interosseous b's of lateral
    terminal b. of deep fibular
    nerve
  interosseous b. of medial
    terminal b. of deep fibular
    nerve
  muscular b's of deep fibu-
    lar nerve
  b. of oculomotor nerve to
    ciliary ganglion

branch *(continued)*
    posterior b's of axillary nerve
    pulmonary b's of vagus nerve, anterior
    pulmonary b's of vagus nerve, posterior
    b's to sternocleidomastoid
    terminal b. of deep fibular nerve, lateral
    terminal b. of deep fibular nerve, medial
    ventral b's of thoracic nerves
    zygomaticofacial b. of zygomatic nerve
    zygomaticotemporal b. of zygomatic nerve

Brauch-Romberg symptom

Bravais-Jacksonian epilepsy

Breschet's sinus

breviradiate

Brill-Zinsser disease

Brissaud
    B's reflex
    B.-Sicard syndrome

Bristowe's syndrome

Broca
    band of B.
    diagonal band of B.
    B's aphasia
    B's center
    B's convolution
    B's diagonal band
    B's fissure
    B's gyrus
    B's motor speech area
    B's parolfactory area
    B's region

Brodmann's areas

Brown
    B.-Roberts-Wells apparatus
    B.-Roberts-Wells technique

Brown *(continued)*
    B.-Vialetto-van Laere syndrome

Brown-Séquard
    B.-S's paralysis
    B.-S's sign
    B.-S's syndrome

Bruce
    tract of B. and Muir
    B's tract

Brudzinski
    B's reflex
    B's sign

Brueghel's syndrome

Bruns
    B's apraxia of gait
    B's frontal ataxia
    B's sign
    B's syndrome

brush
    Ruffini's b.

Brushfield-Wyatt syndrome

bud
    gustatory b.
    taste b.

bulb
    end b.
    end b. of Held
    end b. of Krause
    b. of Krause
    Krause's end b.
    b. of occipital horn of lateral ventricle
    olfactory b.
    onion b.
    b. of posterior horn of lateral ventricle
    terminal b. of Krause

bulbopontine

bulbus
    b. cornus occipitalis ventriculi lateralis
    b. olfactorius

bulbus *(continued)*
    b. cornus posterioris ventriculi lateralis
    b. encephali

bundle
    aberrant b's
    comb b.
    Helweg's b.
    longitudinal medial b.
    medial forebrain b.
    Meynert's b.
    Monakow's b.
    olivocochlear b. of Rasmussen
    b. of Oort
    posterior longitudinal b.
    b. of Rasmussen
    Schütz's b.
    solitary b.
    thalamomammillary b.

bundle *(continued)*
    Türck's b.

Büngner's bands

Burdach
    cuneate fasciculus of B.
    column of B.
    fasciculus of B.
    B's fibers
    B's fissure
    nucleus of B's column

burst

butterfly

button
    terminal b.

bypass
    extracranial/intracranial (EC/IC) b.

C
C fibers

cachinnation

cacodemonomania

cacogeusia

cacosmia

caeruleus

Cajal
horizontal cell of C.
interstitial nucleus of C.
C. cell

calamus
c. scriptorius

calcar
c. avis

calcaroid

calcinosis
cerebral c.

calciorrhachia

caliculus *pl.* caliculi
c. gustatorius

California encephalitis

Calleja
islands of C.
C's islets

callosal

callosomarginal

callosotomy

callosum

campotomy

canal
central c.
central c. of spinal cord
craniopharyngeal c.
supraoptic c.

canalis
c. centralis medullae spinalis

Canavan
C's disease
C.-van Bogaert-Bertrand
disease

Cantelli's sign

Canto-Rapin syndrome

capacitance
membrane c.

capsula *pl.* capsulae
c. externa
c. extrema
c. ganglii
c. interna
c. nuclei dentati
capsulae nuclei lentiformis

capsule
external c.
extreme c.
c. of ganglion
internal c.

caput
c. cornus dorsalis medullae
spinalis
c. cornus posterioris me-
dullae spinalis
c. nuclei caudati

carbamazepine

Carbatrol

Carbidopa

carcinoma *pl.* carcinomas, car-
cinomata
choroid plexus c.
leptomeningeal c.
meningeal c.

carcinomatosis
leptomeningeal c.
meningeal c.

carina *pl.* carinae
c. fornicis

carotidynia

carotodynia

Carpenter
C's syndrome
C.-Philappart syndrome

carpoptosis

caryochrome

cascabel

cat

catalogia

cataphasia

cataplectic

cataplexis

cataplexy

catatonia

catatonic

catecholamine

catecholaminergic

catelectrotonus

catheter
toposcopic c.

cauda *pl.* caudae
c. equina
c. nuclei caudati

caudatolenticular

causalgia

Cavare's disease

cave
Meckel's c.
c. of septum pellucidum
trigeminal c.

cavitas
c. epiduralis
c. septi pellucidi
c. subarachnoidea
c. subarachnoidealis
c. trigeminalis

cavity
epidural c.

cavity *(continued)*
head c.
c. of septum pellucidum
subarachnoid c.
subdural c.
trigeminal c.

cavum *pl.* cava
c. epidurale
c. psalterii
c. septi pellucidi
c. subarachnoideum
c. trigeminale

cavy

Cayler syndrome

Cd

cell
Alzheimer's c's
anterior horn c's
apolar c.
basket c.
Bergmann's c's
Betz's c's
bipolar c.
bipolar retinal c's
breviradiate c's
Cajal c.
capsule c.
caudate c's
chief c's
Clarke's c's
commissural c's
compound granule c.
ependymal c's
epithelioid c's
excitable c.
Fañanás' c.
fatty granule c.
ganglion c.
giant pyramidal c's
Gierke's c's
gitter c.
glial c's
globoid c.
Golgi's c's
granule c's
gustatory c's
hecatomeral c's

cell *(continued)*
- heteromeral c's
- heteromeric c's
- horizontal c. of Cajal
- horn c's
- Hortega c.
- integrator c.
- interstitial c's
- karyochrome c.
- Martinotti's c's
- Mauthner's c.
- Merkel c.
- Merkel tactile c.
- Meynert's c's
- microglia c.
- microglial c.
- mitral c's
- mossy c.
- motor c.
- Nageotte's c's
- nerve c.
- neuroendocrine c's
- neuroepithelial c's
- neuroglia c's
- neuroglial c's
- neurosecretory c.
- olfactory c's
- olfactory receptor c's
- periglomerular c's
- physaliferous c's
- physaliphorous c's
- pineal c.
- Purkinje c's
- pyramidal c.
- Renshaw c's
- rod c's
- Rohon-Beard c's
- Rolando's c's
- root c's
- Sala's c's
- satellite c's
- Schultze's c's
- Schwann c.
- sensory c.
- solitary c's of Meynert
- spider c.
- tactile c.
- taste c's
- tautomeral c's

cell *(continued)*
- touch c.
- tufted c.

cenesthesia

cenesthesic

cenesthetic

cenesthopathy

center
- accelerating c.
- anospinal c's
- apneustic c.
- auditopsychic c.
- Broca's c.
- Budge's c.
- cardioaccelerating c.
- cardioinhibitory c.
- cardiovascular control c's
- ciliospinal c.
- coordination c.
- coughing c.
- defecation c.
- deglutition c.
- ejaculation c.
- erection c.
- eupraxic c.
- feeding c.
- genital c.
- genitospinal c.
- glossokinesthetic c.
- heat-regulating c's
- hunger c.
- Kronecker's c.
- Lumsden's c.
- medullary c.
- medullary c. of cerebellum
- medullary respiratory c.
- micturition c.
- nerve c.
- panting c.
- pneumotaxic c.
- polypneic c.
- rectovesical c.
- reflex c.
- respiratory c's
- satiety c.
- semioval c.
- sensory c's

center *(continued)*
    sex-behavior c.
    sudorific c.
    swallowing c.
    sweat c.
    thermoregulatory c's
    thirst c.
    vasoconstrictor c.
    vasodilator c.
    vasomotor c's
    vesical c.
    vesicospinal c.
    vomiting c.
    word c., auditory

central
    c. canal
    c. canal of spinal cord
    C. European encephalitis

centraphose

centrencephalic

centrophose

centrum *pl.* centra
    c. semiovale

cephalad

cephalalgia
    histamine c.
    pharyngotympanic c.
    quadrantal c.

cephaledema

cephalgia

cephalhematocele
    Stromeyer's c.

cephalhematoma
    c. deformans

cephalhydrocele
    c. traumatica

cephalic

cephalocele
    orbital c.

cephalocentesis

cephalochordate

cephalodynia

cephalogyric

cephalohematocele

cephalohematoma

cephalomotor

cephalopathy

cephaloplegia

cercopithecoid

cerea flexibilitas

cerebella

cerebellar

cerebellifugal

cerebellipetal

cerebellitis

cerebellofugal

cerebello-olivary

cerebellopontile

cerebellopontine

cerebellorubral

cerebellorubrospinal

cerebellospinal

cerebellum

cerebra

cerebral
    c. calcinosis
    c. toxoplasmosis

cerebrifugal

cerebripetal

cerebrocerebellar

cerebrology

cerebromacular

cerebromalacia

cerebromeningeal

cerebromeningitis

cerebropathia
    c. psychica toxemica

cerebropathy

cerebrophysiology

cerebropontile

cerebrorachidian

cerebrosclerosis

cerebrosis

cerebrospinal

cerebrostomy

cerebrotomy

cerebrovascular

cerebrum

Cerebyx

ceruleus

cervical
    c. spondylosis

cervicobrachialgia

cervix
    c. of axon
    c. cornus dorsalis medullae
        spinalis
    c. cornus posterioris me-
        dullae spinalis

CES

Cestan
    C's syndrome
    C.-Chenais syndrome
    C.-Raymond syndrome

Chaddock
    C's reflex
    C's sign

Chagas' disease

chain
    nuclear c.
    sympathetic c.

channel
    PQ calcium c.

Charcot
    C's arthropathy
    C's disease
    C's gait
    C's joint
    C's sign
    C's syndrome
    C's triad
    C.-Marie atrophy
    C.-Marie syndrome
    C.-Marie-Tooth atrophy
    C.-Marie-Tooth disease
    C.-Weiss-Baker syndrome

Charlin's syndrome

Chédiak-Higashi syndrome

cheiralgia
    c. paresthetica

chemoceptor

chemonucleolysis

chemopallidectomy

chemopallidothalamectomy

chemoreception

chemoreceptor

chemosensory

chemothalamectomy

Chiari
    C's deformity
    C's malformation
    C.-Arnold syndrome

chiasm
    optic c.

chiasma *pl.* chiasmata
    optic c.
    c. opticum

chimpanzee

chirobrachialgia

chirognostic

cholesteatoma
    congenital c.
    intracranial c.

cholesteatomatous

cholinergic

cholinoceptive

cholinoceptor

cholinomimetic

chondroskeleton

chorda *pl.* chordae
    c. tympani

chordate

chordoblastoma

chordocarcinoma

chordoepithelioma

chordoma

chordosarcoma

chordotomy

chorea
    acute c.
    chronic c.
    chronic progressive heredi-
      tary c.
    chronic progressive non-
      hereditary c.
    c. cordis
    dancing c.
    degenerative c.
    c. dimidiata
    Dubini's c.
    electric c.
    fibrillary c.
    c. gravidarum
    hemilateral c.
    hereditary c.
    Huntington's c.
    juvenile c.
    methodic c.
    mimetic c.
    c. minor

chorea *(continued)*
    c. nocturna
    c. nutans
    one-sided c.
    paralytic c.
    posthemiplegic c.
    saltatory c.
    senile c.
    simple c.
    Sydenham's c.

choreal

choreic

choreiform

choreoacanthocytosis

choreoathetoid

choreoathetosis
    familial paroxysmal c.
    paroxysmal c.
    paroxysmal kinesigenic c.

choreoid

choriomeningitis
    lymphocytic c.

choroidectomy

Christensen-Krabbe disease

chromatolysis

chromophose

chromosome

chronaxie

chronaxy

chronotaraxis

Churg-Strauss syndrome

Chvostek
    C's sign
    C.-Weiss sign

chymopapain

ciliospinal

cilium

cimbia

cinclisis

cinerea

cinereal

cingula

cingulectomy

cingulotomy

cingulum

cingulumotomy

circle
    arterial c. of Willis
    c. of Willis
    cerebral arterial c.

CircOlectric bed

circuit
    Papez c.
    reflex c.
    reverberating c.

circulation
    hypophysial portal c.
    portal c.
    hypophysioportal c.

circulus *pl.* circuli
    c. arteriosus cerebri
    c. arteriosus [Willisi]
    c. willisii

circumcallosal

circumduction

circumferential branches

circumgemmal

circuminsular

circumventricular

cistern
    ambient c.
    basal c.
    c. of chiasma
    chiasmatic c.
    c. of fossa of Sylvius
    great c.

cistern *(continued)*
    interpeduncular c.
    c. of lateral cerebral fossa
    pontine c.
    posterior c.
    posterior cerebellomedul-
      lary c.
    subarachnoid c's

cisterna *pl.* cisternae
    c. ambiens
    c. basalis
    c. cerebellomedullaris pos-
      terior
    c. chiasmatica
    c. fossae lateralis cerebri
    c. fossae Sylvii
    c. interpeduncularis
    c. magna
    c. mesencephalicum
    c. pontis
    c. retrothalamica
    cisternae subarachnoideae
    c. venae magnae cerebri

cisternal

Clarke
    C's cells
    C's column
    dorsal nucleus of C.
    C's nucleus

classification
    Frankel C.
    International C. of Seizures

Claude
    C's hyperkinesis sign
    C's syndrome

claudication
    neurogenic c.

claustra

claustral

claustrum

clava

claval

clavate

cleft
    branchial c.
    Lanterman's c's
    primary synaptic c.
    Schmidt-Lanterman c's
    secondary synaptic c's
    subneural c's
    synaptic c.

Climara

clivus
    c. monticuli

clonazepam

clonic

clonicity

clonicotonic

clonism

clonismus

clonospasm

clonus
    ankle c.
    foot c.
    patellar c.
    wrist c.

Cloquet
    C's ganglion
    C's pseudoganglion

clouding
    c. of consciousness

clunial

coagulation
    massive c.

Coats' disease

Cobb syndrome

cochleotopic

coccyx

Cockayne syndrome

coefficient
    olfactory c.

coenuriasis

coenurosis

coeruleus

Cogentin

Coffin-Siris syndrome

Cogan
    C's oculomotor apraxia
    C's syndrome

Cognex

cognitive
    c. dysfunction
    c. impairment

collateral
    Schaffer c's

Collet
    C's syndrome
    C.-Sicard syndrome

colliculus pl. colliculi
    caudal c.
    c. caudalis
    c. caudatus
    c. facialis
    c. inferior
    rostral c.
    c. rostralis
    c. superior

collision

colpocephaly

column
    anterior c. of spinal cord
    anterolateral c.
    autonomic c. of spinal cord
    c. of Burdach
    Clarke's c.
    dorsal funicular c.
    dorsal gray c.
    dorsal c. of spinal cord
    fornix c.
    c. of fornix
    fundamental c.
    c. of Goll
    Gowers' c.

column *(continued)*
    gray c's
    gray c. of spinal cord, anterior
    gray c. of spinal cord, lateral
    gray c. of spinal cord, posterior
    intermediate c. of spinal cord
    interomediolateral c. of spinal cord
    lateral c. of spinal cord
    c. of Lissauer
    posterior c. of spinal cord
    posteromedian c. of medulla oblongata
    posteromedian c. of spinal cord
    c. of Spitzka and Lissauer
    Stilling's c.
    striomotor c.
    thoracic c.
    Türck's c.
    ventral c. of spinal cord
    white c's of spinal cord

columna *pl.* columnae
    c. anterior medullae spinalis
    c. autonomica medullae spinalis
    c. dorsalis medullae spinalis
    c. fornicis
    columnae griseae medullae spinalis
    c. intermedia medullae spinalis
    c. intermediolateralis medullae spinalis
    c. lateralis medullae spinalis
    c. posterior medullae spinalis
    c. thoracica
    c. ventralis medullae spinalis

coma
    agrypnodal c.
    alcoholic c.
    alpha c.
    hepatic c.
    c. hepaticum
    irreversible c.
    c. vigil

comatose

commissura *pl.* commissurae
    c. alba anterior medullae spinalis
    c. alba posterior medullae spinalis
    c. anterior
    c. colliculi caudalis
    c. colliculi inferioris
    c. colliculi rostralis
    c. colliculi superioris
    c. epithalamica
    c. fornicis
    c. grisea anterior medullae spinalis
    c. grisea anterior/posterior medullae spinalis
    c. grisea posterior medullae spinalis
    c. habenularum
    c. magna cerebri
    c. olivarum
    c. posterior
    c. rostralis
    c. supraoptica dorsalis
    c. supraoptica ventralis

commissure
    anterior c.
    c. of caudal colliculus
    cerebral c., posterior
    c. of epithalamus
    c. of fornix
    Ganser's c.
    gray c.
    gray c. of spinal cord
    gray c. of spinal cord, anterior
    gray c. of spinal cord, anterior/posterior

commissure *(continued)*
    gray c. of spinal cord, dorsal
    gray c. of spinal cord, posterior
    gray c. of spinal cord, ventral
    Gudden's c.
    c. of habenulae
    habenular c.
    hippocampal c.
    c. of inferior colliculus
    Meynert's c.
    posterior c.
    rostral c.
    c. of rostral colliculus
    c. of superior colliculus
    supraoptic c's
    supraoptic c., dorsal
    supraoptic c., ventral
    white c. of spinal cord, anterior
    white c. of spinal cord, dorsal
    white c. of spinal cord, posterior
    white c. of spinal cord, ventral

commotio
    c. cerebri
    c. spinalis

complex
    AIDS dementia c.
    amygdaloid c.
    calcarine c.
    K c.
    oculomotor nuclear c.
    olivary c., inferior
    olivary c., superior
    perihypoglossal c.
    perihypoglossal nuclear c.
    posterior nuclear c. of thalamus
    ventral lateral c. of thalamus
    ventral medial c. of thalamus
    ventrobasal c. of thalamus

complexus
    c. olivaris inferior

component
    somatic motor c.
    somatic sensory c.
    splanchnic motor c.
    splanchnic sensory c.
    visceral motor c.
    visceral sensory c.

compression
    c. of the brain
    cerebral c.
    nerve c.
    spinal c.
    spinal cord c.

COMT-inhibitor

concha

concrete thinking

concussion
    c. of the brain
    c. of the spinal cord

conduction
    antidromic c.
    avalanche c.
    ephaptic c.
    saltatory c.
    synaptic c.

cone
    bifurcation c.
    cerebellar pressure c.
    growth c.
    implantation c.
    medullary c.
    pressure c.
    terminal c. of spinal cord

coney

confluence
    c. of sinuses

confluens
    c. sinuum

congestion
    neurotonic c.

connexus
  c. interthalamicus

conscious

consciousness

Constantinidis-Wisniewski syndrome

contraction
  clonic c.
  myotatic c.
  paradoxical c.
  tetanic c.
  tonic c.
  twitch c.

contrecoup

control
  idiodynamic c.
  motor c.
  reflex c.
  tonic c.
  volitional c.
  voluntary c.

contusion
  brain c.
  contrecoup c.
  c. of spinal cord

conus *pl.* coni
  c. medullaris
  c. terminalis

convergence
  multimodal c.
  multisensory c.

convolution
  Broca's c.
  c's of cerebrum
  Heschl's c's
  occipitotemporal c.
  Zuckerkandl's c.

convulsant

convulsibility

convulsion
  central c.
  clonic c.

convulsion *(continued)*
  essential c.
  local c.
  mimetic c.
  mimic c.
  salaam c's
  tetanic c.
  tonic c.
  uremic c.

convulsivant

convulsive

coordination

Copaxone

copolymer-1

coprodaeum, coprodeum

coprophagia

coprophagy

cord
  Bergmann's c's
  lateral c. of brachial plexus
  medial c. of brachial plexus
  posterior c. of brachial plexus
  spinal c.
  tethered c.
  Willis' c's

cordectomy

cordotomy
  open c.
  percutaneous c.

Cornelia de Lange's syndrome

cornu *pl.* cornua
  c. ammonis
  c. anterius medullae spinalis
  c. anterius ventriculi lateralis
  c. dorsale medullae spinalis
  c. frontale ventriculi lateralis
  c. inferius ventriculi lateralis

cornu *(continued)*
 c. laterale medullae spinalis
 c. occipitale ventriculi lateralis
 c. posterius medullae spinalis
 c. posterius ventriculi lateralis
 cornua of spinal cord
 c. temporale ventriculi lateralis
 c. ventrale medullae spinalis

cornucommissural

corona
 c. radiata

corpus *pl.* corpora
 c. amygdaloideum
 corpora bigemina
 c. callosum
 c. cerebelli
 c. fimbriatum hippocampi
 c. fornicis
 c. geniculatum laterale
 c. geniculatum mediale
 c. mammillare
 c. medullare cerebelli
 c. nuclei caudati
 c. pineale
 corpora quadrigemina
 c. restiforme
 c. striatum
 c. subthalamicum
 c. trapezoideum

corpuscallosotomy

corpuscle
 articular c.
 axile c.
 axis c.
 bulboid c.
 chorea c's
 chromophil c's
 compound granular c.
 Dogiel's c.
 genital c.
 Gluge's c's

corpuscle *(continued)*
 Golgi's c.
 Golgi-Mazzoni c's
 Herbst's c's
 Krause's c.
 lamellar c.
 lamellated c.
 lingual c.
 Mazzoni's c.
 Meissner's c.
 Merkel's c.
 pacchionian c's
 Pacini's c.
 pacinian c.
 Ruffini's c.
 Schwalbe's c.
 tactile c.
 taste c.
 terminal nerve c.
 Timofeew's c.
 touch c.
 Valentin's c's
 Vater's c.
 Vater-Pacini c.

corpusculum *pl.* corpuscula
 c. articulare
 c. bulboideum
 c. genitale
 c. lamellosum
 c. nervosum terminale
 c. tactus

cortex
 agranular c.
 cerebellar c.
 c. cerebellaris
 c. cerebelli
 c. of cerebellum
 cerebral c.
 c. cerebralis
 c. cerebri
 c. of cerebrum
 granular c.
 heterotypical c.
 homotypical c.
 motor c.
 nonolfactory c.
 olfactory c.
 piriform c.

cortex *(continued)*
  somesthetic c.
  striate c.
  visual c.

Corti's ganglion

corticectomy

corticifugal

corticipetal

corticoafferent

corticoautonomic

corticobulbar

corticodiencephalic

corticoefferent

corticofugal

corticomesencephalic
  c. tract

corticopeduncular

corticopetal

corticopontine

corticopontocerebellar

corticospinal

corticothalamic

Cotard's syndrome

Cotte's operation

Cotugno's disease

Cotunnius
  nerve of C.

cough
  trigeminal c.

Crafts' test

craniamphitomy

craniectomy

craniocele

craniocerebral

craniomeningocele

craniopharyngioma

craniopuncture

craniosacral

craniospinal

craniotome

craniotomy

craniotopography

craniotrypesis

crepuscular

Creutzfeldt
  C.-Jakob disease
  new variant C.-Jakob dis-
    ease

Crichton-Browne's sign

crisis
  bronchial c.
  cardiac c.
  clitoris c.
  gastric c.
  intestinal c.
  laryngeal c.
  myasthenic c.
  nephralgic c.
  oculogyric c.
  parkinsonian c.
  pharyngeal c.
  rectal c.
  renal c.
  tabetic c.
  thoracic c.
  vesical c.
  visceral c.

crispation

cross
  Ranvier's c's
  silver c's

Crouzon's disease

Crow-Fukase syndrome

Crowe's sign

crus *pl.* crura
    c. I
    c. II
    anterior c. of internal capsule
    c. anterius capsulae internae
    c. cerebri
    c. fornicis
    posterior c. of internal capsule
    c. posterius capsulae internae
    c. primum lobuli ansiformis
    c. secundum lobuli ansiformis
    superior c. of cerebellum

Cruveilhier
    C's atrophy
    C's disease
    C's paralysis
    C's plexus

cry
    epileptic c.

cryalgesia

cryanesthesia

cryesthesia

cryoanalgesia

cryohypophysectomy

cryothalamectomy

cryothalamotomy

cryptomerorachischisis

CT
    computed tomography

cuirass
    tabetic c.

culmen
    c. cerebelli
    c. of cerebellum

cuneus *pl.* cunei

current
    action c.
    ascending c.
    centrifugal c.
    centripetal c.
    descending c.
    electrotonic c.
    nerve-action c.

Curschmann-Steinert syndrome

curse
    Ondine's c.

curve
    strength-duration c.

Cushing
    C's disease
    C's phenomenon

cyanophose

cycle
    Hodgkin c.

Cylert

cylinder
    axis c.
    Ruffini's c.
    terminal c.

cynanthropy

cynomolgus

Cyon
    C's experiment
    C's nerve

cyst
    arachnoid c.
    colloid c.
    craniobuccal c's
    craniopharyngeal c's
    ependymal c.
    epidermoid c.
    intrapituitary c's
    leptomeningeal c.
    neural c.
    neurenteric c.
    perineurial c.

cyst *(continued)*
    porencephalic c.
    Rathke's c's
    Rathke's cleft c's
    soapsuds c's
    suprasellar c.
    Tarlov c.

cytodendrite

cytodistal

cyton

cytoproximal

D
    D sleep

daboia

dance
    St. Anthony's d.
    St. Guy's d.
    St. John's d.
    St. Vitus' d.

Dandy
    D's operation
    D.-Walker deformity
    D.-Walker malformation
    D.-Walker syndrome

Dantrium

dantrolene

Darkshevich's nucleus

dassie

Davidenko syndrome

Dawson's encephalitis

deafferentation

deafness
    cortical d.
    music d.
    nerve d.
    neural d.
    perceptive d.
    sensorineural d.
    tone d.
    toxic d.
    word d.

death
    brain d.
    cerebral d.
    cognitive d.

decerebellation

decerebrate

decerebration

decerebrize

de Clérambault syndrome

declive

declivis

decomposition
    d. of movement

decompression
    cerebral d.
    microvascular d.
    nerve d.
    d. of spinal cord
    suboccipital d.
    subtemporal d.

decussatio *pl.* decussationes
    d. fibrarum nervorum tro-
      chlearium
    d. lemnisci medialis
    d. motoria
    d. nervorum trochlearis
    d. nervorum trochlearium
    d. pedunculorum cerebel-
      larium superiorum
    d. pyramidum
    decussationes tegmentales
    d. tegmentalis anterior
    d. tegmentalis posterior
    decussationes tegmenti
    decussationes tegmento-
      rum
    d. trochlearis

decussation
    anterior tegmental d.
    dorsal tegmental d.
    Forel's d.
    fountain d. of Meynert
    d. of medial lemniscus
    motor d.
    optic d.
    posterior tegmental d.
    pyramidal d.
    d. of pyramids
    rubrospinal d.
    sensory d.
    d. of superior cerebellar
      peduncles
    tectospinal d.
    tegmental d's

decussation *(continued)*
    d's of tegmentum
    trochlear d.
    d. of trochlear nerves
    d. of trochlear nerve fibers
    ventral tegmental d.

defatigation

defect
    neural tube d.
    retention d.
    reversible ischemic neurol-
      ogic d. (RIND)

deficiency
    myelin basic protein d.

deficit
    reversible ischemic neurol-
      ogic d.

deformity
    Arnold-Chiari d.
    Chiari's d.
    Dandy-Walker d.

degeneratio
    d. micans

degeneration
    Alzheimer's neurofibril-
      lary d.
    ascending d.
    axonal d.
    cerebellar d., paraneoplas-
      tic
    cerebellar d., paraneoplas-
      tic subacute
    cerebellar d., primary pro-
      gressive
    cerebromacular d.
    cerebroretinal d.
    comma d.
    corticostriatal-spinal d.
    descending d.
    fascicular d.
    glistening d.
    Gombault's d.
    granulovascular d.
    gray d.
    Holmes's d.
    Nissl d.

degeneration *(continued)*
    olivopontocerebellar d.
    pallidal d.
    retrograde d.
    rim d.
    Rosenthal's d.
    secondary d.
    spongy d. of central ner-
      vous system
    spongy d. of white matter
    striatonigral d.
    subacute combined d. of
      spinal cord
    transneuronal d.
    traumatic d.
    Türck's d.
    uratic d.
    vacuolar d.
    wallerian d.
    white matter d.

degustation

deiteral

Deiters
    D's nucleus
    D's process
    D's tract

Dejean's syndrome

Dejerine
    D's disease
    D's sign
    D's syndrome
    D.-Klumpke paralysis
    D.-Klumpke syndrome
    D.-Landouzy dystrophy
    D.-Roussy syndrome
    D.-Sottas atrophy
    D.-Sottas disease
    D.-Sottas neuropathy
    D.-Thomas atrophy
    D.-Thomas syndrome

delirium
    senile d.

dementia
    Alzheimer's d.
    d. of the Alzheimer type
    arteriosclerotic d.

dementia *(continued)*
    Binswanger's d.
    boxer's d.
    dialysis d.
    epileptic d.
    multi-infarct d.
    myoclonic d.
    d. myoclonica
    paralytic d.
    d. paralytica
    posttraumatic d.
    d. praecox
    presenile d.
    d. pugilistica
    senile d.
    subcortical d.
    vascular d.

Demianoff's sign

De Morsier syndrome

demyelinate

demyelination
    segmental d.

demyelinization

dendric

dendrite
    apical d.

dendritic

dendrodendritic

dendron

dendrophagocytosis

denervate

denervation

Dennie-Marfan syndrome

Denny-Brown
    D.-B's sensory neuropathy
    D.-B's sensory radicular
      neuropathy
    D.-B's syndrome

density
    fiber d.

dentatothalamic

dentatum

deoxyribonucleic acid (DNA)

Depakene

Depakote

depolarization

depolarize

depolarizer

depression
    Leão's spreading d.
    postactivation d.
    spreading d.

depressor

derailment

derealization

dermatome

dermatomic

dermatoneurology

dermohygrometer

dermometer

dermometry

dermatomyositis

dermoneurotropic

descendens
    d. cervicalis
    d. cervicis
    d. hypoglossi

desensitize

De Toni-Fanconi syndrome

developmental age

Devic's disease

dextral

dextrality

dextrocerebral

dextromanual

dextropedal

dextrosinistral

DHE 45

diadochocinesia

diadochokinesia

diadochokinesis

diadochokinetic

diaphemetric

diaphragm
    sellar d.
    d. of sella turcica
    splinted d.

diaphragma *pl.* diaphragmata
    d. sellae

diaschisis

Diastat

diastematomyelia

diataxia
    cerebral d.
    d. cerebralis infantilis

diaxon

diazepam

dichroic

dichroism

diencephalic

diencephalohypophysial

diencephalon

DiGeorge syndrome

digitatio *pl.* digitationes
    digitationes hippocampi

Dilantin

3,4-dimethoxyphenylethylamine

diplegia
    atonic-astatic d.
    facial d.

diplegia *(continued)*
    facial d., congenital
    Förster's d.
    masticatory d.
    spastic d.

diplegic

diplomyelia

diplopia

direction
    ventrocaudal d.

dirigomotor

discectomy

discharge
    bizarre high-frequency d.
    bizarre repetitive d.
    complex repetitive d.
    double d.
    epileptic d.
    epileptiform d's
    grouped d.
    iterative d.
    multiple d.
    myokymic d.
    myotonic d.
    nervous d.
    neural d.
    periodic lateralized epilep-
       tiform d.
    repetitive d.
    triple d.

discoidectomy

discopathy
    traumatic d.

disdiadochokinesia

disease
    Addison's d.
    Akureyri d.
    Alexander's d.
    Alpers' d.
    Alzheimer's d.
    Anderson's d.
    anterior horn cell d.
    Aran-Duchenne d.
    Armstrong's d.

disease *(continued)*
    Australian X d.
    autoimmune d.
    Azorean d.
    Baló's d.
    Bamberger's d.
    Batten d.
    Bayle's d.
    Becker's d.
    Behçet d.
    Bernhardt's d.
    Bernhardt-Roth d.
    Bielschowsky d.
    Billroth's d.
    Binswanger's d.
    Blocq's d.
    Bouchet-Gsell d.
    Boehme d.
    Brill-Zinsser d.
    Canavan's d.
    Canavan-van Bogaert-Bertrand d.
    Cavare's d.
    central core d.
    Chagas' d.
    Charcot's d.
    Charcot-Marie-Tooth d.
    Christensen-Krabbe d.
    Coats' d.
    combined system d.
    Cotugno's d.
    Creutzfeldt-Jakob d.
    Creutzfeldt-Jakob d., new variant
    Crouzon's d.
    Cruveilhier's d.
    Cushing's d.
    degenerative d.
    Dejerine's d.
    Dejerine-Sottas d.
    demyelinating d.
    Devic's d.
    Dubini's d.
    Duchenne's d.
    Duchenne-Aran d.
    Duchenne-Griesinger d.
    Economo's d.
    Ehlers-Danlos d.
    Erb's d.

disease *(continued)*
    Erb-Charcot d.
    Erb-Goldflam d.
    Eulenburg's d.
    extrapyramidal d.
    Fabry d.
    Fahr d.
    Farber d.
    Fazio-Londe d.
    Flatau-Schilder d.
    Friedreich's d.
    Gaucher d.
    Gerlier's d.
    Gilles de la Tourette's d.
    Goldflam's d.
    Goldflam-Erb d.
    Greenfield's d.
    Guinon's d.
    Hallervorden-Spatz d.
    Hammond's d.
    Hartnup d.
    Heine-Medin d.
    Hers' d.
    heredodegenerative d.
    Heubner's d.
    Hippel-Lindau d.
    Horton's d.
    Hunt's d.
    Huntington's d.
    Hurst d.
    Jakob's d.
    Jakob-Creutzfeldt d.
    Joseph d.
    jumping d.
    Koshevnikoff's (Koschewnikow's, Kozhevnikov's) d.
    Krabbe's d.
    Kufs' d.
    Lafora's d.
    Lake-Cavanaugh d.
    laughing d.
    Leigh d.
    Lichtheim's d.
    Lindau's d.
    Lindau-von Hippel d.
    Little's d.
    Lou Gehrig d.
    lower motor neuron d.

disease *(continued)*
>Machado-Joseph d.
>Marchiafava-Bignami d.
>Marie-Tooth d.
>Medin's d.
>Merzbacher-Pelizaeus d.
>Minor's d.
>Möbius' d.
>Morton's d.
>motor neuron d.
>motor system d.
>moyamoya d.
>multicore d.
>Murray Valley d.
>Niemann's d.
>Niemann-Pick d.
>Norrie's d.
>Parkinson's d.
>Parrot's d.
>Pelizaeus-Merzbacher d.
>Pick's d.
>Portuguese-Azorean d.
>prion d.
>Recklinghausen's d.
>Refsum d.
>Roth's (Rot's) d.
>Roth-Bernhardt (Rot-Bernhardt) d.
>Schilder's d.
>Scholz's d.
>Seitelberger's d.
>startle d.
>Strümpell's d.
>Strümpell-Leichtenstern d.
>swineherd's d.
>Talma's d.
>Thomsen's d.
>Tooth's d.
>transmissible neurodegenerative d.
>Unverricht's d.
>Univerricht-Lundborg d.
>upper motor neuron d.
>von Economo's d.
>von Hippel-Lindau d.
>von Recklinghausen's d.
>Wartenberg's d.
>Weber's d.
>Werdnig-Hoffmann d.

disease *(continued)*
>Wernicke's d.
>Weston Hurst d.
>white matter degenerative d's
>Whytt's d.
>Wilson's d.
>Ziehen-Oppenheim d.

disequilibrium

disesthesia

disk
>contained d.
>extruded d.
>herniated d.
>intervertebral d's
>Merkel's d.
>noncontained d.
>d. prolapse
>protruded d.
>Ranvier's tactile d's
>ruptured d.
>sequestered d.
>slipped d.
>tactile d.

diskectomy

disorder
>affective d.
>breathing-related sleep d.
>brief psychotic d.
>demyelinating d.
>delusional d.
>d. of consciousness
>dissociated sensory d.
>dysmyelinating/hypomyelinating d's
>formal thought d.
>induced psychotic d.
>neuronal migration d's
>paranoid d.
>periodic limb movement d.
>postconcussional d.
>psychotic d.
>rapid eye movement sleep behavior d.
>REM sleep behavior d.
>schizoaffective d.
>schizophreniform d.

disorder *(continued)*
    seasonal affective d.
    shared psychotic d.
    simple deteriorative d.
    sleep d's
    substance-induced psychotic d.

dispersion
    temporal d.

dissociation
    syringomyelic d.
    tabetic d.

divalproex

divisio *pl.* divisiones
    divisiones anteriores
        plexus brachialis
    d. autonomica systematis
        nervosi peripherici
    divisiones posteriores
        plexus brachialis

division
    anterior d's of brachial
        plexus
    autonomic d. of peripheral
        nervous system
    craniosacral d.
    dorsal d's of trunks of brachial plexus
    mandibular d.
    maxillary d.
    posterior d's of brachial
        plexus
    thoracicolumbar d.
    thoracolumbar d.
    ventral d's of trunks of brachial plexus

Divry-Van Boegart syndrome

dizziness

DNA
    deoxyribonucleic acid

doctrine
    Monro-Kellie d.
    neuron d.

Dogiel's corpuscle

dol

dolor
    d. capitis

dolorific

dolorimeter

dolorimetry

dolorogenic

dominance
    cerebral d.
    lateral d.
    one-sided d.

donepezil

dopamine

dopaminergic

Doppler
    transcranial D.
    transcranial D. B-mode

dorsum *pl.* dorsa
    d. sellae

doublet

Down syndrome

drainage
    basal d.

dream

drivenness
    organic d.

driving
    photic d.

dromotropic

dromotropism
    negative d.
    positive d.

drop
    wrist d.

drug
    antiepileptic d.

drunkenness
    sleep d.

Dubini
    D's chorea
    D's disease

Dubowitz syndrome

Duchenne
    D's disease
    D's dystrophy
    D's muscular dystrophy
    D's paralysis
    D's syndrome
    D. type muscular dystrophy
    D.-Aran disease
    D.-Aran muscular atrophy
    D.-Erb paralysis
    D.-Erb syndrome
    D.-Griesinger disease
    D.-Landouzy dystrophy

Duckworth
    D's phenomenon
    D's sign

Duncan's ventricle

dura

dural

dura mater
    d. m. of brain
    d. m. cranialis
    d. m. encephali
    d. m. of spinal cord
    d. m. spinalis

duraplasty

Duret's hemorrhages

duroarachnitis

Dyke-Davidoff-Masson syndrome

Dyken
    D. syndrome
    D.-Edathodu syndrome
    D.-Wisniewski syndrome

dying-back

dynamogenesis

dynamogenic

dynamogeny

dynamopathic

dynorphin

dysanagnosia

dysantigraphia

dysaphia

dysarthria
    ataxic d.

dysarthric

dysautonomia
    familial d.

dysbasia
    d. lordotica progressiva

dyscalculia

dyschiasia

dyschiria

dyscinesia

dysdiadochocinesia

dysdiadochokinesia

dysdiadochokinetic

dysequilibrium
    dialysis d.

dysergia

dysesthesia

dysesthetic

dysfunction
    cognitive d.

dysgeusia

dysgrammatism

dysgraphia

dyskinesia
    orofacial d.
    tardive d.
    withdrawal-emergent d.

dyskinetic

dyslexia

dysmetria
  ocular d.

dysmnesia

dysmnesic

dysmyelination

dysmyotonia

dysnomia

dysosmia

dysphasia

dysphrasia

dysplasia
  cortical d.

dysponesis

dyspraxia

dysraphia

dysreflexia
  autonomic d.

dysrhythmia
  cerebral d.
  electroencephalographic d.

dyssomnia

dysstasia

dysstatic

dyssymbolia

dyssymboly

dyssynergia
  d. cerebellaris myoclonica
  d. cerebellaris progressiva
  detrusor–external sphinc-
    ter d.
  detrusor-sphincter d.
  detrusor–striated sphinc-
    ter d.
  vesico-sphincter d.

dystasia
  hereditary areflexic d.
  Roussy-Lévy hereditary ar-
    eflexic d.

dystaxia

dystonia
  d. deformans progressiva
  d. lenticularis
  d. musculorum deformans
  oromandibular d.
  tardive d.
  torsion d.

dystonic

dystrophin

dystrophoneurosis

dystrophia
  d. musculorum progressiva

dystrophy
  Becker's muscular d.
  Becker type muscular d.
  Dejerine-Landouzy d.
  distal muscular d.
  Duchenne's d.
  Duchenne's muscular d.
  Duchenne type muscular d.
  Duchenne-Landouzy d.
  Emery-Dreifuss muscular d.
  Erb's d.
  Erb's muscular d.
  facioscapulohumeral mus-
    cular d.
  Fukuyama type congenital
    muscular d.
  Gowers' muscular d.
  infantile neuroaxonal d.
  Landouzy d.
  Landouzy-Dejerine d.
  Landouzy-Dejerine muscu-
    lar d.
  Leyden-Möbius muscular d.
  limb-girdle muscular d.
  muscular d.
  neuraxonal d.
  neuroaxonal d.
  oculopharyngeal d.

dystrophy *(continued)*
    oculopharyngeal muscu-
      lar d.
    pelvifemoral muscular d.
    progressive muscular d.
    pseudohypertrophic mus-
      cular d.

dystrophy *(continued)*
    reflex sympathetic d.
    scapulohumeral muscu-
      lar d.
    scapuloperoneal muscu-
      lar d.
    Simmerlin's d.

E

E
   E wave

Eaton-Lambert syndrome

ecaudate

ecchondrosis
   e. physaliphora

echographia

echolalia

echopraxia

Ecker's fissure

Economo
   E's disease
   E's encephalitis

edema
   brain e.
   cerebral e.
   cytotoxic e.
   interstitial e.
   vasogenic e.

Edinger
   E's fibers
   E's nuclei
   E.-Westphal nuclei

edipism

Edward's syndrome

effect
   clasp-knife e.
   Mierzejewski e.

effector

efferent

Ehlers-Danlos disease

Ehrenritter's ganglion

Eichhorst's atrophy

Ekbom syndrome

Eldepryl

electroanalgesia

electrocontractility

electrocorticogram

electrocorticography

electrode
   bifilar needle e.
   bipolar needle e.
   bipolar stimulating e.
   coaxial needle e.
   concentric needle e.
   exploring e.
   indifferent e.
   monopolar needle e.
   monopolar stimulating e.
   multilead e.
   needle e.
   recording e.
   reference e.
   scalp e.
   stimulating e.
   surface e.

electroencephalogram
   flat e.
   isoelectric e.

electroencephalograph

electroencephalography

electroencephaloscope

electrogram

electrograph

electrography

electrogustometry

electromyography
   single fiber e.

electroneurography

electroneurolysis

electronystagmography

electrophysiologic

electrophysiology

electrospectrogram

electrospectrography

electrospinogram

electrostriatogram

electrotonic

electrotonus

electrovagogram

elephantiasis
  e. neuromatosa

Elsberg's test

embolism
  cerebral e.
  spinal e.

embolus

Emery-Dreifuss muscular dystrophy

eminence
  collateral e. of lateral ven-
    tricle
  facial e. of eminentia teres
  hypoglossal e.
  medial e. of rhomboid
    fossa
  median e.
  postchiasmatic e.
  postfundibular e.
  terete e.
  trigeminal e.

eminentia *pl.* emininentiae
  e. collateralis ventriculi lat-
    eralis
  e. medialis fossae rhomboi-
    deae
  e. teres

emprosthotonos

emprosthotonus

encephalalgia

encephalatrophy

encephalauxe

encephalic

encephalitic

encephalitides

encephalitis
  e. A
  acute disseminated e.
  acute necrotizing e.
  Australian X e.
  e. B
  benign myalgic e.
  Binswanger's e.
  e. C
  California e.
  Central European e.
  chronic subcortical e.
  cytomegalovirus e.
  Dawson's e.
  eastern equine e.
  Economo's e.
  epidemic e.
  e. epidemica
  equine e.
  forest-spring e.
  granulomatous amebic e.
  hemorrhagic e.
  herpes e.
  herpes simplex e.
  herpetic e.
  HIV e.
  Ilheus e.
  influenzal e.
  Japanese e.
  Japanese B e.
  La Crosse e.
  lead e.
  Leichtenstern's e.
  lethargic e.
  e. lethargica
  limbic e.
  microglial nodular e.
  Murray Valley e.
  e. periaxialis concentrica
  e. periaxialis diffusa
  postinfectious e.
  postvaccinal e.
  Powassan e.

encephalitis *(continued)*
   purulent e.
   pyogenic e.
   Russian autumnal e.
   Russian endemic e.
   Russian forest-spring e.
   Russian spring-summer e.
   Russian tick-borne e.
   Russian vernal e.
   St. Louis e.
   Schilder's e.
   Semliki Forest e.
   Strümpell-Leichtenstern e.
   subacute inclusion body e.
   e. subcorticalis chronica
   summer e.
   suppurative e.
   tick-borne e.
   toxoplasmic e.
   van Bogaert's e.
   Venezuelan equine e.
   vernal e.
   vernoestival e.
   Vienna e.
   von Economo's e.
   western equine e.
   West Nile e.
   woodcutter's e.

encephalitogen

encephalitogenic

encephalocele
   basal e.
   frontal e.
   occipital e.

encephaloclastic

encephalocystocele

encephalodialysis

encephaloduroarteriosynan-giosis

encephalodysplasia

encephaloid

encephalolith

encephaloma

encephalomalacia

encephalomeningitis

encephalomeningocele

encephalomeningopathy

encephalometer

encephalomyelitis
   acute disseminated e.
   acute necrotizing hemor-rhagic e.
   autoimmune e.
   eastern equine e.
   equine e.
   postinfectious e.
   postvaccinal e.
   toxoplasmic e.
   Venezuelan equine e.
   viral e.
   virus e.
   western equine e.

encephalomyelocele

encephalomyeloneuropathy

encephalomyelopathy
   postinfection e.
   postvaccinial e.
   subacute necrotizing e.

encephalomyeloradiculitis

encephalomyeloradiculopathy

encephalomyopathy
   mitochondrial e.

encephalon

encephalonarcosis

encephalopathic

encephalopathy
   AIDS e.
   anoxic e.
   autosomal recessive syn-drome of progressive e.
   bilirubin e.
   boxer's e.

encephalopathy *(continued)*
    boxer's traumatic e.
    cytomegalovirus e.
    demyelinating e.
    dialysis e.
    hepatic e.
    HIV e.
    HIV-related e.
    hypernatremic e.
    hypertensive e.
    hypoglycemic e.
    hypoxic e.
    hypoxic-ischemic e.
    Lyme e.
    lead e.
    metabolic e.
    mitochondrial e.
    multicystic e.
    portal-systemic e.
    portasystemic e.
    progressive dialysis e.
    progressive subcortical e.
    punch-drunk e.
    saturnine e.
    static e.
    subacute necrotizing e.
    subacute spongiform e.
    subcortical arteriosclerot-
      ic e.
    transmissible spongiform e.
    traumatic e.
    uremic e.
    Wernicke's e.

encephalopuncture

encephalopyosis

encephalorachidian

encephaloradiculitis

encephalorrhagia
    pericapillary e.

encephalosclerosis

encephaloscope

encephaloscopy

encephalosepsis

encephalosis

encephalospinal

encephalothlipsis

encephalotomy

endarteritis
    Heubner's e.

endbrain

end-brush

end-bulb

end-foot

ending
    annulospiral e's
    club e. of Bartelmez
    encapsulated nerve e.
    epilemmal e's
    flower-spray e's
    free nerve e.
    grape e's
    nerve e's
    nonencapsulated nerve e.
    primary e's
    Ruffini's e.
    secondary e's

end-nuclei

endocranial

endocraniosis

endocranitis

endocranium

endoneural

endoneurial

endoneuritis

endoneurium

endoneurolysis

endoperineuritis

end-organ

endorphin

endothelioma
  dural e.

endotherm

endothermal

endothermic

endothermy

end plate
  motor e. p.

enervation

engram

engraphia

enkephalin

enkephalinergic

enlargement
  cervical e.
  choroidal e.
  lumbar e.
  lumbosacral e.
  tympanic e.

enolase
  neuron-specific e.

enthlasis

entorhinal

entrapment

enzyme

ependopathy

ependyma

ependymal

ependymitis

ependymoblastoma

ependymocyte

ependymocytoma

ependymoma

ependymopathy

ephapse

ephaptic

epicritic

epidermoid

epidermoidoma

epidural

epilemma

epilemmal

epilepsia
  e. partialis continua

epilepsy
  abdominal e.
  absence e.
  acquired e.
  activated e.
  audiogenic e.
  Baltic myoclonic e.
  benign e. with centrotem-
    poral spikes
  benign rolandic e.
  benign e. with rolandic
    spikes
  Bravais-jacksonian e.
  chronic focal e.
  cortical e.
  cryptogenic e.
  diurnal e.
  essential e.
  focal e.
  gelastic e.
  generalized e.
  generalized flexion e.
  grand mal e.
  haut mal e.
  idiopathic e.
  jacksonian e.
  juvenile myoclonic e.
  Koshevnikoff's (Koschewni-
    kow's, Kozhevnikov's) e.
  Lafora's myoclonic e.
  larval e.
  late e.
  latent e.
  localized e.
  major e.

epilepsy *(continued)*
- matutinal e.
- menstrual e.
- minor e.
- minor focal e.
- musicogenic e.
- myoclonic e.
- myoclonus e.
- nocturnal e.
- organic e.
- partial e.
- partial complex e.
- petit mal e.
- photic e.
- photogenic e.
- photosensitive e.
- physiologic e.
- post-traumatic e.
- procursive e.
- progressive myoclonic e.
- progressive familial myoclonic e.
- psychic e.
- psychogenic e.
- psychomotor e.
- reading e.
- reflex e.
- rolandic e.
- rotatory e.
- sensory e.
- somatosensory e.
- symptomatic e.
- tardy e.
- temporal lobe e.
- traumatic e.
- uncinate e.
- vertiginous e.
- video game e.
- visual e.

epileptic

epileptiform

epileptogenesis

epileptogenic

epileptogenous

epileptoid

epileptologist

epileptology

epinephrine

epineurial

epineurium

epiphysiopathy

epiphysis
- e. cerebri

epipia

epipial

episode
- acute schizophrenic e.

episternal

episternum

episthotonos

epitela

epithalamic

epithalamus

epithelium
- sense e.
- sensory e.
- subcapsular e.

epitonic

equilibrium

equivalent
- migraine e.
- psychic e.

Erb
- E's atrophy
- E's disease
- E's dystrophy
- E's muscular dystrophy
- E's palsy
- E's paralysis
- E's sclerosis
- E.-Charcot disease
- E.-Duchenne palsy
- E.-Duchenne paralysis
- E.-Goldflam disease

Erben
  E's phenomenon
  E's reflex
  E's sign

ergoesthesiograph

erotomania

erythrochromia

erythromelalgia
  e. of the head

erythrophose

Escherich
  E's reflex
  E's sign

esthematology

esthesia

esthesic

esthesiodic

esthesiogenic

esthesiology

esthesiometer

esthesioneure

esthesiophysiology

esthesodic

esthetic

état
  é. criblé
  é. lacunaire
  é. marbré

ethosuximide

eugnosia

eugnostic

eukinesia

eukinesis

eukinetic

eulaminate

Eulenburg's disease

eumetria

euosmia

eupractic

eupraxia

eupraxic

eutherian

eversion

exanimation

Excegran

excitability

excitable

excitant

excitation

excitatory

excitement
  catatonic e.

excitomotor

excitomuscular

excitor

excitotoxic

excitotoxicity

excitotoxin

exhaustion
  postactivation e.
  posttetanic e.

Exner's plexus

experiment
  Cyon's e.

exteroceptive

exteroceptor

extracerebral

extracorticospinal

extracranial

extradural

extramedullary

extrameningeal

extrapyramidal

F
  F waves

Fabry disease

facies
  f. inferior cerebri
  f. inferior hemispherii cere-
    belli
  f. inferior hemispherii cere-
    bri
  f. medialis hemispherii cer-
    ebri
  f. medialis et inferior hemi-
    spherii cerebri
  myasthenic f.
  myopathic f.
  Parkinson's f.
  parkinsonian f.
  f. superior hemispherii cer-
    ebelli
  f. superolateralis cerebri
  f. superolateralis hemisphe-
    rii cerebri

facilitation
  postactivation f.
  posttetanic f.
  Wedensky f.

faciocephalalgia

facioplegia

factor
  nerve growth f.

Fahr disease

faint

Fajersztajn's crossed sciatic
  sign

falling-out

Fallopio
  foramen of F.

falsification
  retrospective f.

falx
  f. cerebelli

falx *(continued)*
  f. cerebri
  f. of cerebellum
  f. of cerebrum

Fañanás
  F's cell
  glia of F.

Fanconi syndrome

Farber disease

fascia *pl.* fasciae
  f. of Tarin

fasciculation
  contraction f's

fasciculus *pl.* fasciculi
  f. aberrans of Monakow
  alvear f.
  anterior f. proprius of spi-
    nal cord
  arcuate f.
  f. arcuatus
  f. of Burdach
  cuneate f. of Burdach
  cuneate f. of medulla ob-
    longata
  cuneate f. of spinal cord
  f. cuneatus medullae oblon-
    gatae
  f. cuneatus medullae spina-
    lis
  dorsal f. proprius of spinal
    cord
  dorsolateral f.
  f. dorsolateralis
  f. of Foville
  fronto-occipital f.
  f. of Goll
  Gowers' f.
  gracile f. of medulla oblon-
    gata
  gracile f. of spinal cord
  f. gracilis medullae oblon-
    gatae
  f. gracilis medullae spinalis
  f. interfascicularis

fasciculus *(continued)*

  intersegmental f. of spinal cord, anterior
  intersegmental f. of spinal cord, dorsal
  intersegmental f. of spinal cord, lateral
  intersegmental f. of spinal cord, posterior
  intersegmental f. of spinal cord, ventral
  lateral f. of brachial plexus
  f. lateralis plexus brachialis
  lateral f. proprius of spinal cord
  f. lenticularis
  longitudinal f., dorsal
  longitudinal f., medial
  longitudinal f., posterior
  longitudinal f. of cerebrum, inferior
  longitudinal f. of cerebrum, superior
  longitudinal f. of medulla oblongata, medial
  f. longitudinalis dorsalis
  f. longitudinalis inferior cerebri
  f. longitudinalis medialis
  f. longitudinalis medialis medullae oblongatae
  f. longitudinalis medialis pontis
  f. longitudinalis posterior
  f. longitudinalis superior cerebri
  f. mammillotegmentalis
  f. mammillothalamicus
  medial f. of brachial plexus
  medial prosencephalic f.
  medial telencephalic f.
  f. medialis plexus brachialis
  f. medialis telencephali
  Meynert's f.
  f. of middle cerebellar peduncle, deep
  f. of middle cerebellar peduncle, inferior

fasciculus *(continued)*

  f. of middle cerebellar peduncle, superior
  Monakow's f.
  occipitofrontal f., inferior
  occipitofrontal f., superior
  f. occipitofrontalis inferior
  f. occipitofrontalis superior
  olivocochlear f.
  f. parieto-occipitopontinus
  perforating f.
  posterior f. of brachial plexus
  f. posterior plexus brachialis
  f. proprius anterior medullae spinalis
  f. proprius dorsalis medullae spinalis
  f. proprius lateralis medullae spinalis
  f. proprius posterior medullae spinalis
  posterior f. proprius of spinal cord
  f. proprius ventralis medullae spinalis
  f. prosencephalicus medialis
  pyramidal f. of medulla oblongata
  f. pyramidalis medullae oblongatae
  f. retroflexus
  Schütz's f.
  semilunar f.
  f. semilunaris
  septomarginal f.
  f. septomarginalis
  solitary f.
  subcallosal f.
  f. subcallosus
  f. subthalamicus
  f. sulcomarginalis
  thalamic f.
  f. thalamicus
  thalamomammillary f.
  f. of Türck
  unciform f.

fasciculus *(continued)*
    uncinate f.
    f. uncinatus
    ventral f. proprius of spinal
        cord
    f. of Vicq d'Azyr

fasciola *pl.* fasciolae
    f. cinerea
    f. cinerea cinguli

fastigial

fastigium

fatigue
    stimulation f.

Fazio
    F.-Londe atrophy
    F.-Londe disease

fear
    ictal f.

Felbamate

Felbatol

feltwork
    Kaes' f.

Ferguson-Critchley ataxia

Ferrein's foramen

festinant

festination

fever
    central f.
    cerebrospinal f.
    West Nile f.

fiber
    A f's
    accelerating f's
    accelerator f's
    A delta f's
    adrenergic f's
    afferent f's
    afferent nerve f's
    alpha f's
    aminergic f's
    amygdalofugal f's

fiber *(continued)*
    arcuate f's
    arcuate f's, anterior exter-
        nal
    arcuate f's, dorsal external
    arcuate f's, internal
    arcuate f's, long
    arcuate f's, posterior exter-
        nal
    arcuate f's, short
    arcuate f's, ventral external
    arcuate f's of cerebrum
    association f.
    association f's, long
    association f's, short
    association f's of telen-
        cephalon
    association nerve f.
    augmentor f's
    autonomic f's
    autonomic nerve f's
    autonomic afferent f's
    autonomic efferent f's
    axial f.
    B f's
    bag f.
    Bergmann's f's
    beta f's
    Burdach's f's
    C f's
    cardiac accelerator f's
    cardiac depressor f's
    cardiac pressor f's
    cerebellovestibular f's
    cerebrospinal f's
    chain f.
    cholinergic f's
    climbing f's
    clinging f's
    commissural f.
    commissural f's of telen-
        cephalon
    corticobulbar f's
    corticonuclear f's
    corticopontine f's
    corticoreticular f's
    corticorubral f's
    corticospinal f's
    corticostriate f's

fiber *(continued)*
    corticothalamic f's
    dentatorubral f's
    dentatothalamic f's
    depressor f's
    Edinger's f's
    efferent f's
    efferent nerve f's
    endogenous f's
    exogenous f's
    frontopontine f's
    fusimotor f's
    gamma f's
    geniculostriate f's
    Goll's f's
    Gratiolet's radiating f's
    gray f's
    heterodesmotic f's
    homodesmotic f's
    internuncial f's
    intersegmental f's
    intrafusal f's
    intrasegmental f's
    intrathalamic f's
    longitudinal pontine f's
    Mauthner's f.
    medullated f's
    medullated nerve f's
    Monakow's f's
    moss f's
    mossy f's
    motor f.
    myelinated f's
    myelinated nerve f's
    nerve f.
    neuroglial f.
    nigrostriate f's
    nonmedullated f's
    nonmedullated nerve f's
    nuclear bag f.
    nuclear chain f.
    oblique gastric f's
    occipitopontine f's
    olivocerebellar f's
    pallidofugal f's
    parallel f's
    paraventricular f's
    parietopontine f's
    parietotemporopontine f's

fiber *(continued)*
    peptidergic f's
    periventricular f's
    pilomotor f's
    pontocerebellar f's
    postcommissural f's
    postganglionic f's
    postganglionic nerve f's
    preganglionic f's
    preganglionic nerve f's
    pressor f's
    projection f.
    projection nerve f's
    radicular f's
    ragged red f's
    Rasmussen's nerve f's
    Reissner's f.
    retinothalamic projection f's
    Rosenthal f's
    somatic f's
    somatic afferent f's
    somatic efferent f's
    somatic nerve f's
    Stilling's f's
    f's of stria terminalis
    striatonigral f's
    sudomotor f's
    supraoptic f's
    T f.
    tangential f's
    tangential nerve f's
    temporopontine f's
    tendril f's
    thalamocortical f's
    thalamoparietal f's
    transverse pontine f's
    trigeminothalamic f's
    ultraterminal f.
    unmyelinated f's
    unmyelinated nerve f's
    varicose f's
    vasomotor f's
    visceral f's
    visceral afferent f's
    visceral efferent f's
    visceral nerve f's
    von Monakow's f's

fibra *pl.* fibrae
    fibrae arcuatae cerebri
    fibrae arcuatae externae
        anteriores
    fibrae arcuatae externae
        dorsales
    fibrae arcuatae externae
        posteriores
    fibrae arcuatae externae
        ventrales
    fibrae arcuatae internae
    f. associationis
    fibrae associationis breves
    fibrae associationis longae
    fibrae associationis telence-
        phali
    f. commissuralis
    fibrae commissurales telen-
        cephali
    fibrae corticonucleares
    fibrae corticopontinae
    fibrae corticoreticulares
    fibrae corticorubrales
    fibrae corticospinales
    fibrae corticothalamicae
    fibrae dentatorubrales
    fibrae frontopontinae
    fibrae intrathalamicae
    fibrae paraventriculares
    fibrae paraventriculohypo-
        physiales
    fibrae parietopontinae
    fibrae parietotemporopon-
        tinae
    fibrae periventriculares
    fibrae pontis longitudinales
    fibrae pontis profundae
    fibrae pontis superficiales
    fibrae pontis transversae
    fibrae pontocerebellares
    f. projectionis
    fibrae striae terminalis
    fibrae supraopticae
    fibrae supraopticohypo-
        physiales
    fibrae temporopontinae
    fibrae thalamoparietales

fibril
    nerve f.
    side f. of Golgi

fibrillation

fibroblastoma
    perineural f.

fibroma *pl.* fibromas, fibromata
    f. molluscum

fibroneuroma

fibropituicyte

fibrosis
    root sleeve f.

field
    eye f.
    f's of Forel
    Forel's f's
    frontal eye f.
    f. H
    f. H of Forel
    f. H_1
    f. H_1 of Forel
    f. H_2
    f. H_2 of Forel
    occipital eye f.
    prerubral f.
    tegmental f.
    Wernicke's f.

figure
    fortification f's

filament
    glial f's
    meningeal f.
    f. of meninges
    pial f. of filum terminale
    root f's of spinal nerve
    spinal f.
    terminal f.
    terminal f., dural
    terminal f., external
    terminal f., internal
    terminal f., pial

filament *(continued)*
    terminal f. of spinal dura mater

fillet

filovaricosis

filum *pl.* fila
    fila anastomotica nervi acustici
    f. durae matris spinale
    fila olfactoria
    fila radicularia nervi spinalis
    f. spinale
    f. terminale
    f. terminale durale
    f. terminale internum
    f. terminale externum
    f. terminale piale

fimbria *pl.* fimbriae
    f. hippocampi

finger
    f.-to-f. test
    f.-nose test
    f.-to-nose test
    f. phenomenon
    f.-thumb reflex

fingeragnosia

firing

Finnish type familial amyloid polyneuropathy

Fisher syndrome

fissura *pl.* fissurae
    fissurae cerebelli
    f. choroidea ventriculi lateralis
    f. dorsolateralis cerebelli
    f. horizontalis cerebelli
    f. intercruralis cerebelli
    f. longitudinalis cerebralis
    f. longitudinalis cerebri
    f. mediana anterior medullae oblongatae

fissura *(continued)*
    f. mediana anterior medullae spinalis
    f. mediana ventralis medullae oblongatae
    f. mediana ventralis medullae spinalis
    f. posterolateralis cerebelli
    f. postpyramidalis
    f. preclivalis
    f. prima cerebelli
    f. secunda cerebelli
    f. transversa cerebralis
    f. transversa cerebri

fissure
    adoccipital f.
    amygdaline f.
    basisylvian f.
    f. of Bichat
    branchial f.
    Broca's f.
    Burdach's f.
    calcarine f.
    callosal f.
    callosomarginal f.
    central f.
    cerebellar f's
    cerebral f's
    cerebral f., great
    cerebral f., great transverse
    cerebral f., lateral
    cerebral f., longitudinal
    cerebral f., transverse
    f's of cerebrum
    choroid f.
    choroid f. of lateral ventricle
    collateral f.
    dentate f.
    dorsolateral f. of cerebellum
    Ecker's f.
    entorbital f.
    great f. of cerebrum
    great horizontal f.
    great transverse f. of cerebrum

fissure *(continued)*
    hippocampal f.
    f. of hippocampus
    horizontal f. of cerebellum
    inferofrontal f.
    intercrural f. of cerebellum
    interparietal f.
    lateral f. of cerebrum
    longitudinal f.
    longitudinal f. of cerebel-
        lum
    longitudinal f. of cerebrum
    median f., anterior
    median f., posterior
    median f. of medulla oblon-
        gata, anterior
    median f. of medulla oblon-
        gata, dorsal
    median f. of medulla oblon-
        gata, posterior
    median f. of medulla oblon-
        gata, ventral
    median f. of spinal cord,
        anterior
    median f. of spinal cord,
        dorsal
    median f. of spinal cord,
        posterior
    median f. of spinal cord,
        ventral
    f. of Monro
    Pansch's f.
    parietooccipital f.
    postcentral f.
    postclival f.
    posterolateral f. of cerebel-
        lum
    postlingual f.
    postlunate f.
    postpyramidal f.
    precentral f.
    preclival f.
    precuneal f.
    prepyramidal f.
    presylvian f.
    primary f. of cerebellum
    retrotonsillar f.
    f. of Rolando
    Schwalbe's f.

fissure *(continued)*
    secondary f. of cerebellum
    subfrontal f.
    subtemporal f.
    superfrontal f.
    supertemporal f.
    sylvian f.
    f. of Sylvius
    transtemporal f.
    transverse f. of cerebrum
    transverse occipital f.
    zygal f.

fistula *pl.* fistulae, fistulas
    carotid cavernous f.
    cerebrospinal fluid f.
    craniosinus f.

fit

flap
    bone f.
    liver f.

Flautau
    F's law
    F.-Schilder disease

flattening
    f. of affect

Flechsig
    F's primordial zones
    F's tract

fleece
    f. of Stilling

flexibilitas
    cerea f.

flexibility
    waxy f.

flexion

floccular

flocculus
    accessory f.

floor
    f. of fourth ventricle
    f. of lateral ventricle
    f. of third ventricle

fluid
    cerebrospinal f.
    ventricular f.

focus *pl.* foci
    epileptogenic f.
    epileptogenic f., secondary
    mirror f.

fog
    mental f.

Foix
    F. syndrome
    F.-Alajouanine syndrome

folie
    f. à deux
    f. gémellaire

folium *pl.* folia
    folia cerebelli
    f. vermis

following

fontanelle

foot
    burning feet
    dangle f.
    drop f.
    end f.
    end-f.
    Friedreich f.
    Morton's f.
    pericapillary end f.
    perivascular f.
    sucker f.

footdrop

foramen *pl.* foramina
    f. caecum of medulla oblon-
        gata
    f. caecum medullae oblon-
        gatae
    f. caecum posterius
    f. caecum of Vicq d'Azyr
    f. diaphragmatis [sellae]
    f. of Fallopio
    Ferrein's f.
    interventricular f.

foramen *(continued)*
    f. interventriculare
    jugular f.
    f. jugulare
    f. of Key and Retzius
    lacerate f., posterior
    f. of Luschka
    f. of Magendie
    f. of Monro
    f. of Pacchioni
    pacchionian f.
    Retzius' f.
    Schwalbe's f.
    f. of Vicq d'Azyr

foraminotomy

forceps
    f. anterior
    frontal f.
    f. frontalis
    f. major
    f. minor
    occipital f.
    f. occipitalis
    f. posterior

forebrain

foregilding

Forel
    areas of F.
    F's decussation
    fields of F.
    field H of F.
    field H_1 of F.
    field H_2 of F.

formatio *pl.* formationes
    f. reticularis medullae ob-
        longatae
    f. reticularis medullae spi-
        nalis
    f. reticularis mesencephali
    f. reticularis pedunculi cer-
        ebri
    f. reticularis pontis
    f. reticularis spinalis
    f. reticularis tegmenti pon-
        tis

formatio *(continued)*
    f. reticularis tegmenti mes-
      encephali
    f. reticularis

formation
    coffin f.
    hippocampal f.
    reticular f.
    reticular f. of brainstem
    reticular f. of spinal cord
    spinal reticular f.
    reticular f. of pons
    reticular f. of mesencepha-
      lon
    reticular f. of medulla ob-
      longata

fornix
    f. of brain

Förster
    F's atonic-astatic syndrome
    F's syndrome

fosphenytoin

fossa *pl.* fossae
    f. cerebellaris
    f. cerebralis
    cranial f., anterior
    cranial f., middle
    cranial f., posterior
    f. cranialis anterior
    f. cranialis media
    f. cranialis posterior
    f. cranii anterior
    f. cranii media
    f. cranii posterior
    ethmoid f.
    f. hypophyseos
    f. hypophysialis
    f. interpeduncularis
    jugular f.
    f. jugularis
    f. jugularis ossis temporalis
    olfactory f.
    pituitary f.
    f. rhomboidea
    sellar f.
    suprasphenoidal f.

fossa *(continued)*
    sylvian f.
    f. of Sylvius
    Tarin's f.
    f. temporalis

Foster frame

Foster Kennedy syndrome

Fournier test

fovea *pl.* foveae
    caudal f.
    f. caudalis
    cranial f.
    f. cranialis
    f. of fourth ventricle
    f. inferior
    f. superior

Foville
    fasciculus of F.
    F's syndrome

fracture
    f. by contrecoup
    depressed f.
    depressed skull f.
    gutter f.
    ping-pong f.
    pond f.

frame
    Foster f.
    Stryker f.

Frankel Classification

Fränkel's sign

Frankenhäuser's ganglion

Fraser syndrome

Frazier-Spiller operation

frenulum *pl.* frenula
    f. of cranial medullary ve-
      lum
    f. of rostral medullary ve-
      lum
    f. of superior medullary ve-
      lum
    f. veli medullaris cranialis
    f. veli medullaris rostralis

frenulum *(continued)*
    f. veli medullaris superioris

Frey
    F's hairs
    F's syndrome

Friedmann's vasomotor syndrome

Friderichsen
    F.-Waterhouse syndrome

Friedreich
    F's ataxia
    F's disease
    F. foot
    F's tabes

Fröhlich syndrome

Froin's syndrome

Froment's paper sign

Frommann's lines

Fryns syndrome

Fugl-Meyer assessment

fugue
    epileptic f.

Fukuhara syndrome

Fukuyama
    F's syndrome
    F. type congenital muscular
      dystrophy

fungus *pl.* fungi
    f. of the brain

fungus *(continued)*
    cerebral f.
    f. cerebri

funiculitis

funiculus *pl.* funiculi
    f. anterior medullae spinalis
    cuneate f.
    f. cuneatus [Burdachi]
    f. cuneatus lateralis
    dorsal f. of spinal cord
    f. dorsalis medullae spinalis
    lateral f. of medulla oblongata
    lateral f. of spinal cord
    f. lateralis medullae oblongatae
    f. lateralis medullae spinalis
    funiculi medullae spinalis
    f. posterior medullae spinalis
    f. separans
    funiculi of spinal cord
    ventral f. of spinal cord
    f. ventralis medullae spinalis

Funkenstein test

funnel
    pial f.

furor
    f. epilepticus

fusimotor

G

GABAergic

gabapentin

Gabitril

gait
> ataxic g.
> calcaneus g.
> cerebellar g.
> Charcot's g.
> gluteus medius g., compensated
> double step g.
> drop-foot g.
> dystrophic g.
> equine g.
> festinating g.
> gluteal g.
> gluteus medius g.
> hemiplegic g.
> hip extensor g.
> intermittent double-step g.
> maximus g.
> myopathic g.
> paraplegic spastic g.
> propulsive g.
> quadriceps g.
> scissor g.
> shuffling g.
> spastic g.
> steppage g.
> stuttering g.
> swaying g.
> tabetic g.
> Trendelenburg g.
> waddling g.

Galen
> G's anastomosis
> G's nerve

galvanogustometer

galvanopalpation

gamma-aminobutyric

ganglia (*plural of* ganglion)

ganglial

gangliated

gangliform

gangliitis

gangliocyte

gangliocytoma

ganglioform

ganglioglioma

ganglioglioneuroma

ganglioma

ganglion *pl.* ganglia
> aberrant g.
> accessory ganglia
> Andersch's g.
> ganglia aorticorenalia
> auditory g.
> Auerbach's g.
> g. autonomicum
> ganglia of autonomic plexuses
> basal ganglia
> Bidder's ganglia
> Blandin's g.
> Bochdalek's g.
> Bock's g.
> ganglia cardiaca
> carotid g.
> caudal g. of glossopharyngeal nerve
> caudal g. of vagus nerve
> g. caudalis nervi glossopharyngei
> g. caudalis nervi vagi
> celiac ganglia
> ganglia celiaca
> cerebrospinal ganglia
> cervical g., inferior
> cervical g., middle
> cervical g., superior
> cervical g. of uterus
> g. cervicale inferioris
> g. cervicale medium
> g. cervicale superius
> g. cervicothoracicum
> cervicouterine g.
> g. ciliare

ganglion *(continued)*
   Cloquet's g.
   g. cochleare
   ganglia coeliaca
   collateral ganglia
   Corti's g.
   cranial sensory g.
   g. craniospinale sensorium
   dorsal root g.
   Ehrenritter's g.
   ganglia encephalica
   encephalospinal g.
   g. encephalospinale
   false g.
   first thoracic g.
   Frankenhäuser's g.
   gasserian g.
   geniculate g.
   g. geniculatum nervi facialis
   g. geniculi nervi facialis
   glossopharyngeal ganglia
   hepatic g.
   hypogastric ganglia
   ganglia of glossopharyngeal nerve
   g. impar
   inferior g. of glossopharyngeal nerve
   inferior g. of vagus nerve
   g. inferius nervi glossopharyngei
   g. inferius nervi vagi
   inhibitory g.
   ganglia intermedia
   jugular g. of glossopharyngeal nerve
   jugular g. of vagus nerve
   Laumonier's g.
   Lee's g.
   lesser g. of Meckel
   Lobstein's g.
   lower g. of glossopharyngeal nerve
   Ludwig's g.
   ganglia lumbalia
   ganglia lumbaria
   Meckel's g.
   Meissner's g.

ganglion *(continued)*
   mesenteric g., inferior
   mesenteric g., superior
   g. mesentericum inferius
   g. mesentericum superius
   g. of Müller
   nerve g.
   g. nervi splanchnici
   neural g.
   nodose g.
   g. oticum
   parasympathetic g.
   g. parasympatheticum
   g. parasympathicum
   ganglia pelvica
   ganglia pelvina
   petrosal g.
   petrosal g., inferior
   petrous g.
   ganglia phrenica
   ganglia plexuum autonomicorum
   ganglia plexuum visceralium
   prevertebral ganglia
   g. pterygopalatinum
   Remak's g.
   ganglia renalia
   Ribes' g.
   rostral g. of glossopharyngeal nerve
   rostral g. of vagus nerve
   g. rostralis nervi glossopharyngei
   g. rostralis nervi vagi
   ganglia sacralia
   Scarpa's g.
   Schmiedel's g.
   semilunar g.
   g. sensoriale
   g. sensorium nervi cranialis
   g. sensorium nervi spinalis
   sensory g.
   sensory g. of cranial nerve
   sensory g. of encephalic nerve
   sphenomaxillary g.
   sphenopalatine g.
   spinal g.

ganglion *(continued)*
    g. spinale
    spiral g.
    g. spirale cochleae
    splanchnic g.
    stellate g.
    g. stellatum
    g. sublinguale
    g. submandibulare
    splanchnic thoracic g.
    g. splanchnicum
    superior g. of glossopha-
      ryngeal nerve
    superior g. of vagus nerve
    g. superius nervi glosso-
      pharyngei
    g. superius nervi vagi
    suprarenal g.
    ganglia of sympathetic
      trunk
    g. sympatheticum
    g. sympathicum
    spiral g. of cochlea
    spiral g. of cochlear nerve
    g. terminale
    ganglia thoracalia
    ganglia thoracica
    g. thoracicum splanchni-
      cum
    g. of trigeminal nerve
    g. trigeminale
    ganglia trunci sympathetici
    tympanic g.
    tympanic g. of Valentin
    ganglia trunci sympathici
    g. tympanicum
    vagal g., inferior
    vagal g., superior
    Valentin's g.
    ventricular ganglia
    g. vertebrale
    g. vestibulare
    visceral g.
    ganglia of visceral plexuses
    g. viscerale

ganglionated

ganglioneuroblastoma

ganglioneurofibroma

ganglioneuroma

ganglionic

ganglionitis
    gasserian g.

gangliosympathectomy

Ganser's commissure

Garcin's syndrome

gargalanesthesia

gargalesthesia

gargalesthetic

Gaucher disease

gegenhalten

Geigel's reflex

Gélineau's syndrome

gemästete

gemistocyte

gemistocytic

gemma
    g. gustatoria

gemmule

generator
    pattern g.

geniculocalcarine

geniculostriate

geniculum *pl.* genicula
    g. nervi facialis

Gennari
    band of G.
    line of G.
    stripe of G.

genu *pl.* genua
    g. capsulae internae
    g. corporis callosi
    g. of facial nerve
    g. of facial nerve, internal
    g. of internal capsule

genu *(continued)*
   g. nervi facialis

Gerlier's disease

germinoma
   pineal g.

Gerstmann
   G's syndrome
   G.-Sträussler syndrome
   G.-Sträussler-Scheinker syn-
      drome

Giacomini's band

giddiness

Gierke's cells

gigantism

Gilles de la Tourette
   G. d. l. T's disease
   G. d. l. T's syndrome

girdle
   Hitzig's g.

gland
   hemal g's
   pineal g.
   pituitary g.

glandula *pl.* glandulae
   g. pinealis
   g. pituitaria

Glasgow
   G. Coma Scale
   G. Outcome Scale

glia
   ameboid g.
   Bergmann's g.
   cytoplasmic g.
   g. of Fañanás
   fibrillary g.

gliacyte

glial

glioblastoma
   g. multiforme

gliocyte

gliofibrillary

glioma
   astrocytic g.
   ependymal g.
   ganglionic g.
   mixed g.
   optic g.
   peripheral g.

gliomatosis
   cerebral g.
   g. cerebri

gliomatous

glioneuroma

gliophagia

gliopil

gliosarcoma

gliosis
   diffuse g.
   hemispheric g.
   hypertrophic nodular g.
   isomorphic g.
   perivascular g.
   unilateral g.

gliosome

globi *(plural of* globus*)*

globule
   Marchi's g's

globulus *pl.* globuli

globus *pl.* globi
   g. pallidus
   g. pallidus lateralis
   g. pallidus medialis
   g. pallidus external seg-
      ment
   g. pallidus internal segment

glomerulus *pl.* glomeruli
   nonencapsulated nerve g.
   olfactory g.
   synaptic g.

glomus *pl.* glomera
   g. choroideum

glossocinesthetic

glossokinesthetic

glossolalia

glossospasm

gluciphore

glucophore

Gluge's corpuscles

glutamate

glutamic acid

glycine

Goebel syndrome

Goldberg-Shprintzen syndrome

Goldenhar
    G's syndrome
    G.-Gorlin syndrome

Goldflam
    G's disease
    G.-Erb disease

Goldthwait's sign

Golgi
    G's cells
    G's corpuscle
    side fibril of G.
    G. tendon organ
    G's theory
    G. type I neurons
    G. type II neurons
    G.-Mazzoni corpuscles

Goll
    column of G.
    fasciculus of G.
    G's fibers
    nucleus of G's column
    G's tract

Gombault
    G's degeneration
    G's neuritis
    G.-Philippe triangle

gomitoli

Gordon
    G's reflex
    G's sign

Gowers
    G's column
    G's fasciculus
    G's maneuver
    G's muscular dystrophy
    G's phenomenon
    G's sign
    G's syndrome
    G's tract

graft
    cable g.
    fascicular g.
    nerve g.
    sleeve g.

grand mal

Granit loop

granulatio *pl.* granulationes
    granulationes arachnoideae
    granulationes arachnoide-
      ales
    granulationes cerebrales

granulation
    arachnoid g's
    arachnoidal g's
    cerebral g's
    pacchionian g's
    Virchow's g's

granule
    chromatic g's
    chromophilic g's
    meningeal g's
    Nissl's g's

granuloma
    malarial g.

graphesthesia

graphomotor

graphorrhea

Grasset
G's phenomenon
G's sign
G.-Bychowski sign
G.-Gaussel phenomenon
G.-Gaussel-Hoover sign

Gratiolet
radiation of G.
G's radiating fibers

Greenfield's disease

Greig syndrome

grippe
g. aurique

groove
anterolateral g. of medulla
oblongata
anterolateral g. of spinal
cord
anteromedian g. of medulla
oblongata
anteromedian g. of spinal
cord
basilar g.
greater petrosal g.
g. for greater petrosal
nerve
g. for lesser petrosal nerve
olfactory g.
posterolateral g. of medulla
oblongata
posterolateral g. of spinal
cord
retroolivary g.

groundhog

group
dorsal respiratory g.
glucophore g.
osmophore g.
sapophore g.
ventral respiratory g.

gryochrome

guanophore

Gubler
G's hemiplegia
G's paralysis

Gudden
G's commissure
G's law

Guillain-Barré
G.-B. polyneuritis
G.-B. syndrome

Guilland's sign

Guinon
G's disease
tic de G.

Gunn
G's phenomenon
G's sign
G's syndrome

gustation

gustometer

gustometry

gyrectomy
frontal g.

gyrencephalic

gyri (*plural of* gyrus)

gyrometer

gyrospasm

gyrus *pl.* gyri
g. angularis
annectant gyri
gyri annectentes
ascending parietal g.
gyri breves insulae
Broca's g.
callosal g.
central g., anterior
central g., posterior
g. cerebelli
gyri cerebri
cingulate g.
g. cinguli

gyrus *(continued)*
g. callosus
cerebral gyri
gyri cerebrales
gyri of cerebrum
g. cingulatus
dentate g.
g. dentatus
g. descendens
g. fasciolaris
g. fornicatus
frontal g., ascending
frontal g., inferior
frontal g., medial
frontal g., middle
frontal g., superior
g. frontalis inferior
g. frontalis medialis
g. frontalis medius
g. frontalis superior
g. fusiformis
g. geniculi
Heschl's gyri
hippocampal g.
g. hippocampi
infracalcarine g.
gyri insulae
interlocking gyri
intralimbic g.
g. lingualis
g. longus insulae
marginal g.
marginal g. of Turner
g. marginalis
occipital gyri, lateral
occipital g., inferior
occipital g., superior
occipitotemporal g., lateral
occipitotemporal g., medial
g. occipitotemporalis lateralis

gyrus *(continued)*
g. occipitotemporalis medialis
g. olfactorius lateralis
g. olfactorius medialis
olfactory g., lateral
olfactory g., medial
gyri orbitales
paracentral g.
g. paracentralis
g. parahippocampalis
g. paraterminalis
parietal g.
g. postcentralis
g. precentralis
preinsular gyri
g. rectus
short gyri of insula
splenial g.
straight g.
subcallosal g.
supracallosal g.
g. supramarginalis
temporal g., anterior transverse
temporal g., inferior
temporal g., middle
temporal g., posterior transverse
temporal g., superior
temporal gyri, transverse
g. temporalis inferior
g. temporalis medius
g. temporalis superior
gyri temporales transversi
g. temporalis transversus anterior
g. temporalis transversus posterior
gyri transitivi cerebri
uncinate g.

H
    H waves

habenula
    h. conarii

habenulae

habu

Haenel symptom

Hahn's sign

hair
    Frey's h's
    gustatory h's
    olfactory h's
    sensory h's
    taste h's

Hakim's syndrome

Haldol

Hallervorden
    H.-Spatz disease
    H.-Spatz syndrome

Hallpike-Bárány positioning maneuver

hallucination
    auditory h.
    olfactory h.
    stump h.
    tactile h.
    visual h.

Hammond's disease

hand
    benediction h.
    drop h.
    Marinesco's succulent h.
    monkey h.
    obstetrician's h.
    phantom h.
    preacher's h.
    writing h.

handedness
    left h.
    right h.

haphalgesia

haptic

haptics

haptometer

harlequin

Hartel's treatment

Harting bodies

Hartley-Krause operation

Hartnup disease

haut mal

head
    h. of caudate nucleus
    h. of dorsal horn of spinal cord
    h. of posterior horn of spinal cord

headache
    alcohol-induced h.
    analgesic rebound h.
    anemic h.
    benign sexual h.
    bilious h.
    blind h.
    carbon monoxide–induced h.
    cluster h.
    congestive h.
    cough h.
    dynamite h.
    ergotamine-induced h.
    exertional h.
    functional h.
    helmet h.
    high-altitude h.
    histamine h.
    Horton's h.
    hyperemic h.
    ice cream h.
    ice-pick pain h.
    lumbar puncture h.
    migraine h.

headache *(continued)*
    monosodium glutamate–induced h.
    nitrate/nitride-induced h.
    organic h.
    postcoital h.
    postspinal h.
    post-traumatic h.
    puncture h.
    pyrexial h.
    reflex h.
    sick h.
    spinal h.
    spondylotic h.
    swim-goggle h.
    symptomatic h.
    tension h.
    tension-type h.
    toxic h.
    vasomotor h.

hearing loss
    sensorineural h. l.

heart
    lymph h.

hebephrenia

hebephrenic

hebetude

hecatomeral

hecatomeric

heel
    h.-knee test
    h.-knee-shin test
    h.-tap test

Heidenhain's syndrome

Heilbronner
    H's sign
    H's thigh

Heine-Medin disease

Held
    end bulb of H.

Heller's syndrome

Helweg
    H's bundle
    H's tract

hemangioblastoma
    cerebellar h.
    spinal h.

hemangioblastomatosis

hemangioendothelioma
    vertebral h.

hematencephalon

hematoencephalic

hematoma
    epidural h.
    parenchymatous h.
    subdural h.

hematomyelia

hematomyelitis

hematomyelopore

hematorrhachis

hemiageusia

hemiageustia

hemialgia

hemiamyosthenia

hemianalgesia

hemianesthesia
    alternate h.
    cerebral h.
    crossed h.
    h. cruciata
    mesocephalic h.
    pontile h.
    spinal h.

hemianosmia

hemiapraxia

hemiasomatognosia

hemiasynergia

hemiataxia

hemiataxy

hemiathetosis

hemiballism

hemiballismus

hemicerebrum

hemichorea

hemicorticectomy

hemicrania
    chronic paroxysmal h.

hemicraniectomy

hemicraniosis

hemicraniotomy

hemidecortication

hemidysergia

hemidysesthesia

hemiepilepsy

hemigeusia

hemihypalgesia

hemihyperesthesia

hemihypermetria

hemihypertonia

hemihypesthesia

hemihypoesthesia

hemihypometria

hemihypotonia

hemi-inattention

hemineglect

hemiopalgia

hemiparalysis

hemiparaplegia

hemiparesis

hemiparesthesia

hemiparetic

hemiparkinsonism

hemiplegia
    h. alternans hypoglossica
    alternate h.
    ascending h.
    capsular h.
    cerebral h.
    contralateral h.
    crossed h.
    h. cruciata
    facial h.
    faciobrachial h.
    faciolingual h.
    flaccid h.
    Gubler's h.
    infantile h.
    spastic h.
    spinal h.
    Wernicke-Mann h.

hemiplegic

hemirachischisis

hemiseptum
    h. cerebri

hemispasm

hemisphaerium

hemisphere
    cerebellar h.
    cerebral h.
    dominant h.
    nondominant h.

hemispherectomy

hemispherium
    h. cerebelli
    h. cerebralis
    h. cerebri

hemitetany

hemithermoanesthesia

hemitonia

hemitremor

hemivagotony

hemorrhachis

hemorrhage
    brain h.
    capsuloganglionic h.
    cerebral h.
    Duret's h's
    extradural h.
    intracerebral h.
    intracranial h.
    intramedullary h.
    intraventricular h.
    parenchymatous h.
    subarachnoid h.
    subdural h.

Henle
    sheath of H.

Herbst's corpuscles

heredoataxia

heredodegeneration

Hering
    H's law
    H's nerve

hernia
    cerebral h.
    h. cerebri
    tonsillar h.

herniation
    caudal transtentorial h.
    disk h.
    h. of intervertebral disk
    h. of nucleus pulposus
    tentorial h.
    tonsillar h.
    transtentorial h.
    uncal h.

herpes
    h. ophthalmicus
    h. zoster auricularis
    h. zoster ophthalmicus
    h. zoster oticus

Herring bodies

Hers' disease

hersage

Heschl
    H's convolutions
    H's gyri

heteresthesia

heterodesmotic

heteroganglionic

heterogeusia

heteromeral

heteromeric

heteromerous

heteropathy

heteropodal

heterosmia

heterotonia

heterotonic

Heubner
    H's disease
    H's endarteritis

hiatus
    h. of canal for greater petrosal nerve
    h. of canal for lesser petrosal nerve
    h. canalis facialis
    h. canalis nervi petrosi majoris
    h. canalis nervi petrosi minoris
    esophageal h.
    h. esophageus
    h. of facial canal
    h. of fallopian canal
    h. fallopii
    false h. of fallopian canal
    h. for greater petrosal nerve
    h. for lesser petrosal nerve
    h. oesophageus
    tentorial h.

hiccup
    epidemic h's

Hick's syndrome

hillock
    axon h.

hilum *pl.* hila
    h. of caudal olivary nucleus
    h. of dentate nucleus
    h. nuclei dentati
    h. of inferior olivary nu-
        cleus
    h. nuclei olivaris caudalis
    h. nuclei olivaris inferioris

hindbrain

Hippel-Lindau disease

hippocampal

hippocampus

Hirano bodies

Hirschberg
    H's reflex
    H's sign

historrhexis

Hitzelberger's sign

Hitzig's girdle

HIV
    human immunodeficiency
        virus (infection)
            HIV encephalitis
            HIV encephalopathy
            HIV-related encepha-
                lopathy

Hochsinger
    H's phenomenon
    H's sign

Hodgkin cycle

Hoffman-Werdnig syndrome

Hoffmann
    H's atrophy
    H's phenomenon

Hoffmann *(continued)*
    H's reflex
    H's sign

hole
    bur h.

Holmes
    H's degeneration
    H's phenomenon
    H's sign
    H.-Adie syndrome
    H.-Stewart phenomenon

holoprosencephaly

holorachischisis

Homén's syndrome

homeotherm

homeothermal

homeothermic

homeothermism

homeothermy

hominid

hominoid

homodesmotic

homoiopodal

homonymous muscle

Hoover's sign

hormone
    adrenocorticotropic h.
        (ACTH)

horn
    horn of Ammon
    anterior horn of lateral
        ventricle
    anterior horn of spinal
        cord
    dorsal horn of spinal cord
    frontal horn of lateral ven-
        tricle
    gray horns of spinal cord
    inferior horn of lateral ven-
        tricle

horn *(continued)*
  lateral horn of spinal cord
  occipital horn of lateral
    ventricle
  posterior horn of lateral
    ventricle
  posterior horn of spinal
    cord
  temporal horn of lateral
    ventricle
  ventral horn of spinal cord
Horner
  H's ptosis
  H's syndrome
  H.-Bernard syndrome
Horsley
  H's operation
  H's sign
Hortega cell
Horton
  H's disease
  H's headache
  H's syndrome
Hughes' reflex
Hunt
  juvenile paralysis agitans
    (of H.)
  H's atrophy
  H's disease
  H's neuralgia
  H's paradoxical phenome-
    non
  H's syndrome
Hunter
  H. syndrome
  H.-McAlpine syndrome
Huntington
  H's chorea
  H's disease
  H's sign
Hurler syndrome
Hutchinson
  H's mask
Hutchison syndrome

Hurst disease
hydranencephaly
hydrencephalocele
hydrencephalomeningocele
Hydrergine
  H. LC
hydroadipsia
hydrocele
  h. spinalis
hydrocephalic
hydrocephalocele
hydrocephaloid
hydrocephalus
  acquired h.
  communicating h.
  congenital h.
  h. ex vacuo
  noncommunicating h.
  normal-pressure h.
  normal-pressure occult h.
  obstructive h.
  occult normal-pressure h.
  otitic h.
  posthemorrhagic h.
  primary h.
  secondary h.
  tension h.
hydrocephaly
hydrodipsomania
hydroencephalocele
hydromeningitis
hydromeningocele
hydromyelia
hydromyelocele
hydromyelomeningocele
hydrophorograph
hydrorachis
hydrosyringomyelia

5-hydroxyindoleacetic acid

5-hydroxytryptamine

3-hydroxytyramine

hygroma
   subdural h.

hypalgesia

hypalgesic

hypalgetic

hypalgia

hypanakinesia

hypanakinesis

hyperacusis

hyperactive

hyperactivity

hyperalgesia
   muscular h.

hyperalgesic

hyperalgetic

hyperalgia

hyperammonemia
   cerebroatrophic h.

hyperanacinesia

hyperanakinesia

hyperaphia

hyperaphic

hyperarousal

hypercinesia

hypercryalgesia

hypercryesthesia

hyperdynamia

hyperdynamic

hyperequilibrium

hyperesthesia
   cerebral h.

hyperesthesia *(continued)*
   gustatory h.
   muscular h.
   olfactory h.
   oneiric h.
   tactile h.

hyperesthetic

hyperexplexia

hypergeusesthesia

hypergeusia

hypergnosis

hyperisotonia

hyperkinesia

hyperkinesis

hyperkinetic

hypermetamorphosis

hypermetria

hypermyotonia

hypernatremia
   hypodipsic h.

hyperosmia

hyperosphresia

hyperpallesthesia

hyperpathia

hyperpolarization

hyperponesis

hyperponetic

hyperpraxia

hyperpselaphesia

hyperreactive

hyperreactivity

hyperreflexia
   autonomic h.
   detrusor h.

hyperresponsive

hyperresponsiveness

hypersensibility

hypersensitive

hypersomnia

hypersomnolence

hypersympathicotonus

hypertarachia

hypertension
    benign intracranial h.
    intracranial h.

hyperthermalgesia

hyperthermesthesia

hyperthermoesthesia

hypertonia

hypertonic

hypertonicity

hypertonus

hypertrophy
    pseudomuscular h.

hyperventilation

hypesthesia

hypnagogic

hypnalgia

hypnocinematograph

hypoalgesia

hypocinesia

hypoequilibrium

hypoergic

hypoesthesia
    gustatory h.
    olfactory h.
    tactile h.

hypoesthetic

hypogeusesthesia

hypogeusia

hypokinesia

hypokinesis

hypokinetic

hypolemmal

hypometria

hypomyelination
    childhood ataxia with cere-
    bral h.

hypopallesthesia

hypophyseal

hypophysectomize

hypophysectomy

hypophyseoportal

hypophysial

hypophysioportal

hypophysis
    h. cerebri

hypophysitis
    lymphocytic h.

hypoponesis

hypopotentia

hypopraxia

hypopselaphesia

hyporeactive

hyporeflexia

hyposensitive

hyposensitivity

hyposmia

hyposomnia

hyposympathicotonus

hyposynergia

hypotension
    chronic orthostatic h.

hypotension *(continued)*
 chronic idiopathic orthostatic h.
 idiopathic orthostatic h.

hypothalamic

hypothalamotomy

hypothalamus

hypothesis
 biogenic amine h.
 gate h.
 jelly roll h.

hypotonia

hypotonic

hypotonus

hypoventilation
 primary alveolar h.

hypsarrhythmia

hypsarrhythmia

hypsokinesis

I
    I substance

ibotenic acid

ibuprofen

ictal

ictus
    i. epilepticus
    i. paralyticus
    i. sanguinis

identification
    cosmic i.

ideomotion

ideomotor

idioglossia

idioglottic

idiolalia

idioreflex

idiospasm

IFN
    interferon
        IFN beta-1

Iggo receptor

Ilheus encephalitis

imaging
    diffusion-weighted i.
    functional magnetic resonance i.
    magnetic resonance i. (MRI)
    magnetic source i.

imbalance
    autonomic i.
    sympathetic i.
    vasomotor i.

Imitrex

impairment
    age-associated memory i.

impairment *(continued)*
    age-related memory i.
    cognitive i.

imperception

implantation
    nerve i.

impressio *pl.* impressiones
    impressiones digitatae
    impressiones gyrorum
    i. petrosa pallii
    i. trigeminalis ossis temporalis
    i. trigemini ossis temporalis

impression
    i's of cerebral gyri
    digital i's
    digitate i's
    gyrate i's bone
    i's of gyri
    trigeminal i. of temporal bone

impulse
    ectopic i.
    nerve i.
    neural i.

inactivator
    electrocerebral i.

inattention
    selective i.

incisura *pl.* incisurae
    i. cerebelli anterior
    i. cerebelli posterior
    i. jugularis ossis occipitalis
    i. jugularis ossis temporalis
    i. preoccipitalis
    i. tentorii cerebelli
    i. of tentorium of cerebellum

incisure
    jugular i. of occipital bone
    jugular i. of temporal bone
    i's of Lanterman
    Lanterman-Schmidt i's
    preoccipital i.

incisure *(continued)*
    Schmidt-Lanterman i's
    temporal i.
    i. of tentorium of cerebellum

incoordination

Inderal
    I. LA

index
    cephalorachidian i.
    cerebrospinal i.
    cephalorhachidian i.

Indiana type familial amyloid polyneuropathy

indicophose

induction
    spinal i.

indusium griseum

infarct
    lacunar i.

infarction
    cerebral i.
    cortical i.
    forebrain i.
    lacunar i.
    migrainous i.
    watershed i.

infranuclear

infratentorial

infundibula *(plural of* infundibulum)

infundibuloma

infundibulum *pl.* infundibula
    i. of hypophysis
    i. hypothalami
    i. of hypothalamus
    i. lobi posterioris hypophyseos
    i. neurohypophyseos

inhibition
    Wedensky i.

inhibitor
    COMT-i.

injection
    intrathecal i.

injury
    whiplash i.

innervation
    double i.
    reciprocal i.

insectivore

insensible

insomnia
    fatal familial i.
    initial i.
    middle i.
    terminal i.

insomniac

insomnic

insufficiency
    basilar i.
    vertebrobasilar i.

insufflation
    cranial i.

insula
    i. of Reil

intention

interbrain

intercentral

intercerebral

interclinoid

interferon (IFN)
    i. beta-1

interganglionic

intergranular

intergyral

interhemicerebral

interhemispheric

interictal

intermeningeal

International Classification of Seizures

interneuron

internode
  i. of Ranvier

internuncial

interoceptive

interoceptor

interolivary

interparoxysmal

interpial

interval
  lucid i.

intra-arachnoid

intracephalic

intracerebellar

intracerebral

intracranial

intradural

intrafissural

intragyral

intraictal

intramedullary

intrameningeal

intraneural

intraparietal

intrapial

intrapontine

intrarachidian

intrasellar

intraspinal

intravertebral

intumescentia *pl.* intumescentiae
  i. cervicalis
  i. lumbalis
  i. lumbosacralis
  i. tympanica

inventory
  Minnesota Multiphasic Personality I. (MMPI)

ionophose

Iowa type familial amyloid polyneuropathy

involuntomotory

ipsilateral

iridocyte

irradiation

irritability
  chemical i.
  electric i.
  mechanical i.
  nervous i.
  specific i.

Isaacs
  I's syndrome
  I.-Mertens syndrome

ischemia
  cerebral i.
  vertebrobasilar i.

ischogyria

island
  i's of Calleja
  olfactory i's
  i. of Reil

islet
  Calleja's i's

isocortex

isothermognosis

isthmus
  i. of cingulate gyrus
  i. gyri cingulatus
  i. gyri cinguli
  i. gyri fornicati
  i. of limbic lobe

iter
  i. ad infundibulum
  i. of Sylvius
  i. e tertio ad quartum ven-
    triculum

Jackson
    J's law
    J's rule
    J's syndrome
    J.-Weiss syndrome

Jacobson's nerve

Jacod
    J's syndrome
    J's triad

Jahnke's syndrome

Jakob
    J's disease
    J.-Creutzfeldt disease

Jamaica
    J. ginger paralysis
    J. ginger polyneuritis

Janet's test

Janz syndrome

Japanese
    J. B encephalitis
    J. encephalitis
    J. type familial amyloid
        polyneuropathy

jararaca

jargonaphasia

Jefferson's syndrome

Jendrassik's maneuver

jerk
    Achilles j.
    ankle j.
    biceps j.
    crossed adductor j.
    elbow j.
    hypnic j's
    jaw j.
    knee j.
    quadriceps j.
    tendon j.
    triceps surae j.

jessur

Joffroy's reflex

Johanson-Blizzard syndrome

joint
    Charcot's j.

Joseph disease

Joubert's syndrome

jugum *pl.* juga
    juga cerebralia

jumping

junction
    myoneural j.
    neuromuscular j.

Juster reflex

juxtallocortex

K
    K complex

Kaes
    K.'s feltwork
    line of K.
    K.'s stria
    K.-Bekhterev layer
    K.-Bekhterev stria

Kahler's law

kainic acid

Kahler's law

kakosmia

Kallmann syndrome

karyochrome

Kearns-Sayre syndrome

Keen's point

Kehrer's reflex

Kennedy's syndrome

Keppra

kernicterus

Kernig's sign

Kernohan's notch

Kerr's sign

Kety-Schmidt method

Key
    foramen of K. and Retzius
    sheath of K. and Retzius

Kienböck's phenomenon

Kiloh-Nevin syndrome

kinanesthesia

kindling

kinesi-esthesiometer

kinesioneurosis

kinesthesia

kinesthesiometer

kinesthesis

kinesthetic

kinohapt

Klein-Levin syndrome

Kleist's sign

Klippel
    K.-Feil syndrome
    K.-Trenaunay-Weber syndrome
    K.-Weil sign

Klonopin

Klumpke
    K's palsy
    K's paralysis
    K.-Dejerine paralysis
    K.-Dejerine syndrome

Klüver-Bucy syndrome

knee
    k. of internal capsule

knife
    gamma k.
    photon k.

knismogenic

knob
    olfactory k.
    synaptic k.

Kocher
    K's point
    K's reflex

Koerber-Salus-Elschnig syndrome

koniocortex

Körte-Ballance operation

Koshevnikoff (Koschewnikow, Kozhevnikov)
    K's disease
    K's epilepsy

Krabbe
    K's disease
    K's leukodystrophy

Krause
    bulb of K.
    K's corpuscle
    end bulb of K.
    K's operation
    terminal bulb of K.

Kronecker's center

kubisagari

Kufs' disease

Kugelberg-Welander syndrome

Kühne's terminal plates

Kuhnt's intermediary tissue

Kurtzke score

kuru

Kussmaul
    K's paralysis
    K.-Landry paralysis

kymatism

labiochorea

labium *pl.* labia
l. cerebri

La Crosse encephalitis

lacuna *pl.* lacunae
cerebral lacunae
lacunae laterales
parasinusoidal lacunae

lacune

Lafora
L's bodies
L's disease
L's myoclonic epilepsy
L's sign

Lake-Cavanaugh disease

Lambert
L.-Eaton myasthenic syndrome
L.-Eaton syndrome

lamella *pl.* lamellae
triangular l.

Lamictal

lamina *pl.* laminae
l. I
l. II
l. III
l. IV
l. V
l. VI
l. affixa
laminae albae cerebelli
laminae corticis cerebri
l. epithelialis
l. granularis externa
l. granularis interna
l. medullaris externa corporis striati
l. medullaris interna corporis striati
l. medullaris lateralis corporis striati
l. medullaris lateralis thalami

lamina *(continued)*
l. medullaris medialis corporis striati
l. medullaris medialis thalami
l. medullaris thalami externa
l. medullaris thalami interna
medullary l. of corpus striatum, external
medullary l. of corpus striatum, internal
medullary l. of corpus striatum, lateral
medullary l. of corpus striatum, medial
medullary l. of thalamus, external
medullary l. of thalamus, internal
l. molecularis
l. multiformis
periclaustral l.
l. plexiformis corticis cerebri
l. pyramidalis externa
l. pyramidalis ganglionaris
l. pyramidalis interna
l. quadrigemina
Rexed's laminae
l. rostralis
l. septi pellucidi
spinal laminae
laminae spinales
l. tectalis mesencephali
l. tecti mesencephali
l. terminalis hypothalami
white laminae of cerebellum

lamotrigine

Lanci
stria of L.

lancinating

Lancisi
longitudinal nerves of L.

89

Lancisi *(continued)*
    nerves of L.

Landau-Kleffner syndrome

Landouzy
    L. dystrophy
    L.-Dejerine atrophy
    L.-Dejerine dystrophy
    L.-Dejerine muscular dystrophy

Landry
    L's paralysis
    L's syndrome

Langer-Giedion syndrome

Langley's nerves

Lanterman
    L's clefts
    incisures of L.
    L.-Schmidt incisures

Leão's spreading depression

Larodopa

laryngismus

laryngoparalysis

laryngoplegia

laryngospasm

Lasègue's sign

latah

latency
    l. of activation
    distal l.
    motor l.
    proximal l.
    REM l.
    residual l.
    sensory l.
    sleep l.
    terminal l.

laterality
    crossed l.
    dominant l.

laughter

Laumonier's ganglion

law
    all-or-none l.
    Bastian's l.
    Bastian-Bruns l.
    Bowditch's l.
    Flatau's l.
    Gudden's l.
    Hering's l.
    Jackson's l.
    Kahler's l.
    Prévost's l.
    l. of reciprocal innervation
    l. of referred pain
    Schroeder van der Kolk's l.
    Sherrington's l.
    van der Kolk's l.

layer
    Bechterew's (Bekhterev's) l.
    l's of cerebral cortex
    fusiform l. of cerebral cortex
    ganglionic l. of cerebellum
    ganglionic l. of cerebral cortex
    glomerular l.
    granular l. of cerebellum
    granular l. of cerebral cortex, external
    granular l. of cerebral cortex, internal
    granular l. of olfactory bulb, external
    granular l. of olfactory bulb, internal
    granule l. of cerebellum
    gray l. of superior colliculus, deep
    gray l. of superior colliculus, intermediate
    gray l. of superior colliculus, superficial
    gray and white l's of rostral colliculus
    gray and white l's of superior colliculus

layer *(continued)*
    Kaes-Bekhterev l.
    medullary l. of thalamus, external
    medullary l. of thalamus, internal
    Meynert's l.
    mitral cell l.
    molecular l. of cerebellum
    molecular l. of cerebral cortex
    molecular l. of olfactory bulb
    multiform l. of cerebral cortex
    nuclear l. of cerebellum
    olfactory nerve fiber l.
    optic l. of superior colliculus
    oriens l. of hippocampus
    peripheral l. of cerebral cortex
    piriform neuronal l.
    plexiform l. of cerebellum
    plexiform l. of cerebral cortex
    polymorphic l. of cerebral cortex
    Purkinje l.
    Purkinje cell l.
    pyramidal l. of cerebral cortex, external
    pyramidal l. of cerebral cortex, internal
    pyramidal l. of hippocampus
    radiate l. of hippocampus
    subcallosal l.
    l's of superior colliculus
    white l's of cerebellum
    white l. of superior colliculus, deep
    white l. of superior colliculus, intermediate
    zonal l. of cerebral cortex
    zonal l. of superior colliculus
    zonal l. of thalamus
Ledbänder

Lee's ganglion

left-handed

leg
    restless l's

leiasthenia

Leichtenstern
    L's phenomenon
    L's sign

Leigh
    L. disease
    L. syndrome

leiodystonia

Leksell
    L. apparatus
    L. technique

Lemieux-Neemeh syndrome

lemnisci

lemniscus
    l. lateralis
    l. medialis
    sensory l.
    l. spinalis
    l. trigeminalis

lemur

Lennox
    L. syndrome
    L.-Gastaut syndrome

lens
    crossed l.

lenticula

lenticular

lenticulo-optic

lenticulostriate

lenticulothalamic

leptomeningeal

leptomeninges

leptomeningioma

leptomeningitis
  sarcomatous l.

leptomeningopathy

leptomeninx

Léri's sign

lesion
  central l.
  local l.
  peripheral l.
  ring-wall l.

lesionectomy

lethargy

leucotomy

leu-enkephalin

leukencephalitis

leukodystrophy
  globoid cell l.
  hereditary adult-onset l.
  hereditary cerebral l.
  Krabbe's l.
  metachromatic l.
  spongiform l.
  sudanophilic l.

leukoencephalitis
  acute hemorrhagic l.
  acute hemorrhagic l. of
    Weston Hurst
  l. periaxialis concentrica
  van Bogaert's sclerosing l.

leukoencephalopathy
  metachromatic l.
  necrotizing l.
  progressive multifocal l.
  subacute sclerosing l.

leukoencephaly

leukomalacia
  periventricular l.

leukomyelitis

leukomyelopathy

leukotome

leukotomy
  transorbital l.

level
  l's of consciousness

Lévy-Roussy syndrome

Lewy bodies

Leyden
  L.-Möbius muscular dystro-
    phy
  L.-Möbius syndrome

Lhermitte's sign

Lichtheim
  L's disease
  L. plaques
  L's syndrome

Liepmann's apraxia

ligament
  coccygeal l.
  dentate l. of spinal cord
  denticulate l.

ligamentum *pl.* ligamenta
  l. denticulatum

limb
  anterior l. of internal cap-
    sule
  inferior l. of ansa cervicalis
  posterior l. of internal cap-
    sule
  phantom l.
  retrolenticular l. of internal
    capsule
  retrolentiform l. of internal
    capsule
  sublenticular l. of internal
    capsule
  sublentiform l. of internal
    capsule
  superior l. of ansa cervi-
    calis

limbic

limen *pl.* limina
    l. insulae
    l. of twoness

liminal

liminometer

limp

Lindau
    L.'s disease
    L.'s tumor
    L.-von Hippel disease

Linder
    L.'s sign
    L.'s test

line
    Baillarger's external l.
    Baillarger's inner l.
    Baillarger's internal l.
    Baillarger's outer l.
    choroid l.
    external l. of Baillarger
    Frommann's l's
    l. of Gennari
    inner l. of Baillarger
    internal l. of Baillarger
    intraperiod l's
    l. of Kaes
    major dense l's
    major period l's
    outer l. of Baillarger
    period l's

linea *pl.* lineae
    l. splendens

lingula *pl.* lingulae
    l. cerebelli

Lioresal

lipidosis
    galactosylceramide l.
    sphingomyelin l.
    sulfatide l.

lipofuscinosis
    ceroid-l.
    neuronal ceroid-l.

lipohyalinotic

lipoma
    epidural l.
    intradural l.
    intramedullary l.
    intraspinal l.

lipomeningocele

lipomyelomeningocele

lipophilin

liquor
    l. cerebrospinalis

Lisch nodules

Lissauer
    column of L.
    L.'s marginal zone
    L.'s paralysis
    L.'s tract

lissencephalia

lissencephalic

lissencephaly
    Walker's l.

Little's disease

Livierato's sign

lobe
    anterior l. of cerebellum
    caudal l. of cerebellum
    cerebral l's
    cranial l. of cerebellum
    cuneate l.
    flocculonodular l.
    frontal l.
    limbic l.
    middle l. of cerebellum
    neural l.
    neural l. of neurohypo-
      physis
    neural l. of pituitary gland
    occipital l.
    olfactory l.
    optic l's
    parietal l.

lobe *(continued)*
    piriform l.
    posterior l. of cerebellum
    posterior l. of hypophysis
    posterior l. of pituitary
      gland
    quadrate l. of cerebral
      hemisphere
    rostral l. of cerebellum
    semilunar l., inferior
    semilunar l., superior
    temporal l.
    vagal l.
    visceral l.

lobectomy
    occipital l.
    temporal l.

lobotomy
    frontal l.
    prefrontal l.
    transorbital l.

Lobstein's ganglion

lobule
    ansiform l.
    biventral l.
    central l. of cerebellum
    gracile l. of cerebellum
    paracentral l.
    paramedian l.
    parietal l., inferior
    parietal l., superior
    quadrangular l. of cerebel-
      lum, anterior
    quadrangular l. of cerebel-
      lum, posterior
    semilunar l., caudal
    semilunar l., cranial
    semilunar l., inferior
    semilunar l., rostral
    semilunar l., superior
    simple l. of cerebellum

lobulus *pl.* lobuli
    l. ansiformis
    l. biventer
    l. centralis cerebelli
    l. gracilis cerebelli

lobulus *(continued)*
    l. paracentralis
    l. paramedianus cerebelli
    l. parietalis inferior
    l. parietalis superior
    l. quadrangularis anterior
      cerebelli
    l. quadrangularis posterior
      cerebelli
    lobuli semilunares
    l. semilunaris caudalis
    l. semilunaris inferior
    l. semilunaris rostralis
    l. semilunaris superior
    l. simplex cerebelli

lobus *pl.* lobi
    l. anterior cerebelli
    l. caudalis cerebelli
    l. cerebelli anterior
    l. cerebelli posterior
    lobi cerebrales
    lobi cerebri
    l. cranialis cerebelli
    l. flocculonodularis
    l. frontalis
    l. insularis
    l. limbicus
    l. nervosus neurohypophy-
      seos
    l. occipitalis
    l. parietalis
    l. posterior cerebelli
    l. posterior hypophysis
    l. rostralis cerebelli
    l. temporalis
    l. vagi

localization
    cerebral l.

lockjaw

locomotion
    brachial l.

locus *pl.* loci
    l. caeruleus
    l. ceruleus
    l. cinereus
    l. coeruleus

locus *(continued)*
    l. ferrugineus

logagraphia

loop
    gamma l.
    Granit l.
    l. of hypoglossal nerve
    Hyrtl's l.
    lenticular l.
    Meyer's l.
    Meyer-Archambault l.
    peduncular l.
    l's of spinal nerves
    subclavian l.
    l. of Vieussens

loosening
    l. of associations

Lou Gehrig disease

Louis-Bar's syndrome

Lovén reflex

Lowe syndrome

Löwenthal's tract

Lowry-MacLean syndrome

Luciani
    triad of L.

Ludwig
    L's ganglion
    L's nerve

Luschka
    foramen of L.
    nerve of L.

Lust
    L's phenomenon
    L's reflex
    L's sign

Luys
    L's body
    nucleus of L.

Lyell's syndrome

lymphoma
    primary central nervous
        system l.

lymphopathy
    ataxic l.

lyra
    l. Davidis

M
> M response

McCarthy's reflex

McCormac's reflex

Macewen's sign

Machado-Joseph disease

Mackenzie's syndrome

macrencephalia

macrencephaly

macrocrania

macroencephaly

macroesthesia

macroglia

macrographia

macrography

macrogyria

macrostereognosia

macula *pl.* maculae
> cerebral m.

maculocerebral

Maffucci's syndrome

Magendie
> foramen of M.
> M's spaces

Magnan's movement

magnetoencephalograph

magnetometer

Magnus and de Kleijn neck re-
flexes

main
> m. d'accoucheur
> m. en singe
> m. succulente

mal
> grand m.

mal *(continued)*
> haut m.
> petit m.

malacia
> m. traumatica

Malacarne's pyramid

maladie
> m. des tics

malformation
> Arnold-Chiari m.
> arteriovenous m. (AVM)
> auditory arteriovenous m.
> cerebral arteriovenous m.
> Chiari's m.
> Dandy-Walker m.

malingering

malleation

maneuver
> Adson's m.
> Allen's m.
> Bárány's m.
> Gowers' m.
> Hallpike-Bárány position-
> ing m.
> Jendrassik's m.
> Phalen's m.
> Schreiber's m.

mantle
> brain m.

march
> cortical m.
> epileptic m.
> jacksonian m.

marche
> m. à petits pas

Marchi
> M's globules
> M's reaction
> M's tract

Marchiafava-Bignami disease

Marcus Gunn
> M. G's phenomenon

Marcus Gunn *(continued)*
    M. G's syndrome

margaritoma

margin
    inferolateral m. of cerebral
      hemisphere
    inferomedial m. of cerebral
      hemisphere
    superior m. of cerebral
      hemisphere
    superomedial m. of cere-
      bral hemisphere

margo
    m. inferior cerebri
    m. inferolateralis hemi-
      spherii cerebri
    m. inferomedialis hemi-
      spherii cerebri
    m. medialis cerebri
    m. superior hemispherii
      cerebri
    m. superomedialis cerebri

Marie
    M's quadrilateral space
    M.-Foix sign
    M.-Tooth disease

Marinesco
    M's sign
    M's succulent hand
    M.-Radovici reflex

marrow
    spinal m.

Martinotti's cells

Maryland type familial amyloid
  polyneuropathy

mask
    Hutchinson's m.
    Parkinson's m.
    tabetic m.

mass
    tigroid m's

massa *pl.* massae
    m. intermedia

Matas' treatment

mater
    arachnoidea m.
    dura m.
    pia m.

Mauthner
    M's cell
    M's fiber
    M's membrane
    M's sheath

matter
    gray m. of nervous system
    white m. of nervous system

Maxalt

Mayer's reflex

Mazzoni's corpuscle

Mebaral

mechanicoreceptor

mechanics
    animal m.

mechanoceptor

mechanoreceptor
    high-threshold m.

mechanosensory

Meckel
    M's cave
    lesser ganglion of M.
    M's ganglion
    M's space

meclizine

mediation
    chemical m.

mediator

medication
    antagonist m.

Medin's disease

medulla
    m. oblongata

medulla *(continued)*
    m. spinalis

medullary

medullated

medullation

medullitis

medulloblastoma

medulloepithelioma

megalencephalon

megalencephaly

megalographia

megalography

megalomania

megalomaniac

Meige's syndrome

Meissner
    M's corpuscle
    M's ganglion
    M's plexus

melanophore

melanophorin

MELAS syndrome

Melkersson-Rosenthal syndrome

Melnick-Fraser syndrome

membrana *pl.* membranae
    m. limitans

membrane
    arachnoid m.
    endoneural m.
    Mauthner's m.
    postsynaptic m.
    presynaptic m.
    Schwann's m.
    synaptic m.

Mendel
    M's dorsal reflex of foot
    M's reflex

Mendel *(continued)*
    M.-Bekhterev reflex
    M.-Bekhterev sign

Meniere's syndrome

meningeal

meningematoma

meningocortical

meningioma

meningiorrhaphy

meninges

meninghematoma

meningioma
    angioblastic m.
    cerebellopontine angle m.
    clival m.
    convexity m's
    cystic m.
    falcine m.
    falx m.
    fibroblastic m.
    fibrous m.
    meningotheliomatous m.
    m. of the olfactory groove
    parasagittal m.
    posterior fossa m.
    psammomatous m.
    m. of the sphenoid ridge
    suprasellar m.
    syncytial m.
    tentorial m.
    transitional m.
    m. of the tuberculum sellae

meningiomatosis

meningism

meningismus

meningitic

meningitides

meningitis
    acute aseptic m.
    aseptic m.
    bacterial m.

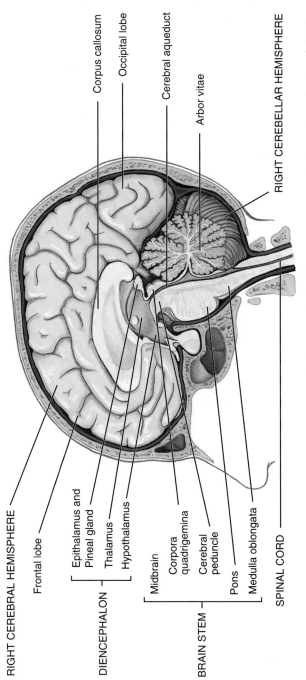

RIGHT CEREBRAL HEMISPHERE

Frontal lobe

DIENCEPHALON
- Epithalamus and Pineal gland
- Thalamus
- Hypothalamus

BRAIN STEM
- Midbrain
  - Corpora quadrigemina
  - Cerebral peduncle
- Pons
- Medulla oblongata

SPINAL CORD

Corpus callosum

Occipital lobe

Cerebral aqueduct

Arbor vitae

RIGHT CEREBELLAR HEMISPHERE

Midsagittal section of the brain showing the major portions of the diencephalon, brain stem, and cerebellum. (From Applegate, E: The Anatomy and Physiology Learning System, 2nd ed. Philadelphia, W. B. Saunders Company, 2000.)

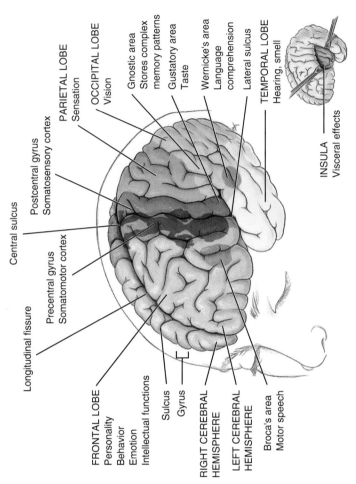

Central sulcus

Longitudinal fissure

Postcentral gyrus
Somatosensory cortex

PARIETAL LOBE
Sensation

OCCIPITAL LOBE
Vision

Gnostic area
Stores complex
memory patterns

Gustatory area
Taste

Wernicke's area
Language
comprehension

Lateral sulcus

TEMPORAL LOBE
Hearing, smell

Precentral gyrus
Somatomotor cortex

INSULA
Visceral effects

FRONTAL LOBE
Personality
Behavior
Emotion
Intellectual functions

Sulcus
Gyrus

RIGHT CEREBRAL
HEMISPHERE

LEFT CEREBRAL
HEMISPHERE

Broca's area
Motor speech

Lobes and functional areas of the cerebellum. (From Applegate, E: The Anatomy and Physiology Learning System, 2nd ed. Philadelphia, W. B. Saunders Company, 2000.)

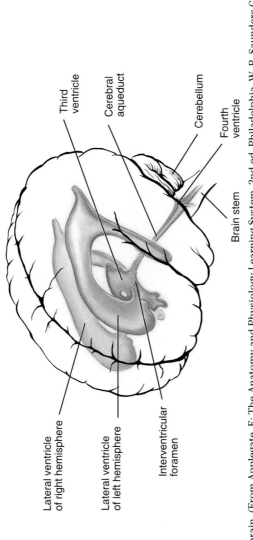

Ventricles of the brain. (From Applegate, E: The Anatomy and Physiology Learning System, 2nd ed. Philadelphia, W. B. Saunders Company, 2000.)

Third ventricle

Cerebral aqueduct

Cerebellum

Fourth ventricle

Brain stem

Lateral ventricle of right hemisphere

Lateral ventricle of left hemisphere

Interventricular foramen

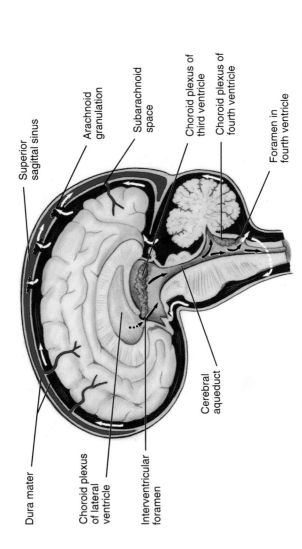

Superior
sagittal sinus

Arachnoid
granulation

Subarachnoid
space

Choroid plexus
of third ventricle

Choroid plexus
of fourth ventricle

Foramen in
fourth ventricle

Dura mater

Choroid plexus
of lateral
ventricle

Interventricular
foramen

Cerebral
aqueduct

Circulation of cerebrospinal fluid. (From Applegate, E: The Anatomy and Physiology Learning System, 2nd ed. Philadelphia, W. B. Saunders Company, 2000.)

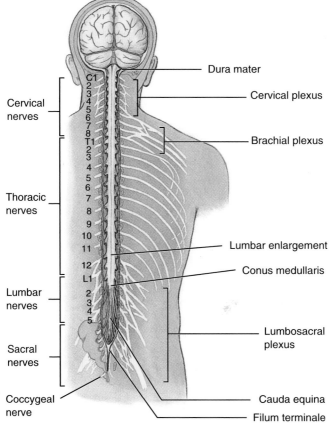

Cervical nerves

Thoracic nerves

Lumbar nerves

Sacral nerves

Coccygeal nerve

C1
2
3
4
5
6
7
8
T1
2
3
4
5
6
7
8
9
10
11
12
L1
2
3
4
5

Dura mater

Cervical plexus

Brachial plexus

Lumbar enlargement

Conus medullaris

Lumbosacral plexus

Cauda equina

Filum terminale

Gross anatomy of the spinal cord. (From Applegate, E: The Anatomy and Physiology Learning System, 2nd ed. Philadelphia, W. B. Saunders Company, 2000.)

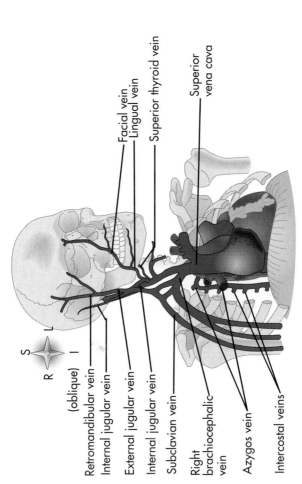

Anterior view showing major veins of the right side of the head and neck. (From Thibodeau, GA, Patton, KT: Anatomy & Physiology, 4th ed. St. Louis, Mosby, Inc. 1999.)

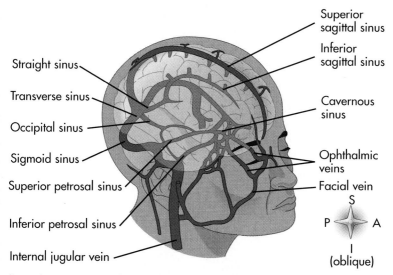

Straight sinus

Transverse sinus

Occipital sinus

Sigmoid sinus

Superior petrosal sinus

Inferior petrosal sinus

Internal jugular vein

Superior sagittal sinus

Inferior sagittal sinus

Cavernous sinus

Ophthalmic veins

Facial vein

S
P A
I
(oblique)

Lateral superior view showing the position of the major veins of the head and neck relative to the brain. (From Thibodeau, GA, Patton, KT: Anatomy & Physiology, 4th ed. St. Louis, Mosby, Inc. 1999.)

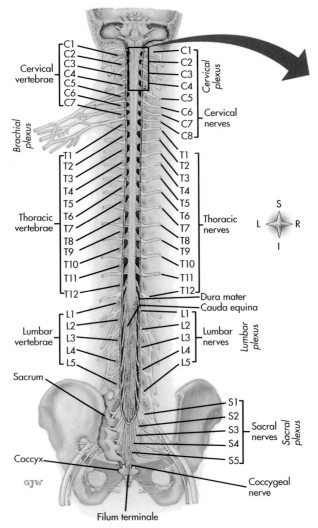

Spinal nerves. Each of 31 pairs of spinal nerves exits the spinal cavity from the intervertebral foramina. The names of the vertebrae are given on the left and the names of the corresponding spinal nerves on the right. Notice that after leaving the spinal cavity, many of the spinal nerves interconnect to form networks called plexuses. (From Thibodeau, GA, Patton, KT: Anatomy & Physiology, 4th ed. St. Louis, Mosby, Inc. 1999.)

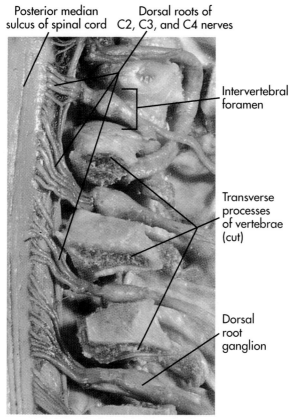

Posterior median sulcus of spinal cord

Dorsal roots of C2, C3, and C4 nerves

Intervertebral foramen

Transverse processes of vertebrae (cut)

Dorsal root ganglion

Dissection of the cervical region, showing a posterior view of cervical spinal nerves exiting intervertebral foramina on the right side. (From Thibodeau, GA, Patton, KT: Anatomy & Physiology, 4th ed. St. Louis, Mosby, Inc. 1999.)

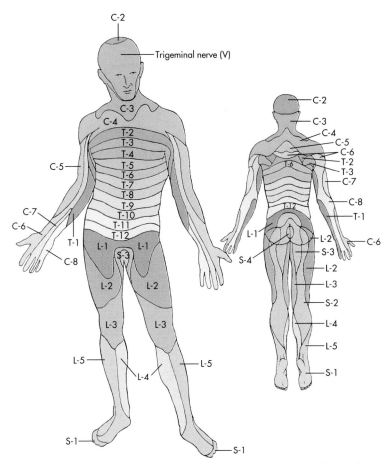

A, Segmental distribution of spinal nerves to front of body. C, Cervical segments; T, thoracic segments; L, lumbar segments; S, sacral segments. *B*, Segmental distribution of spinal nerves to back of the body. (From Applegate, E: The Anatomy and Physiology Learning System, 2nd ed. Philadelphia, W. B. Saunders Company, 2000.)

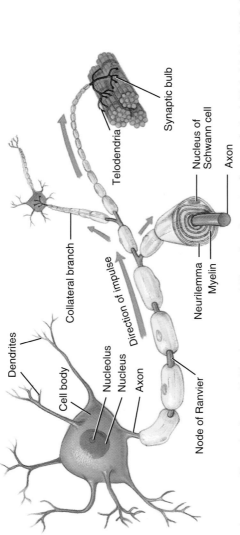

Structure of a typical neuron. (From Applegate, E: The Anatomy and Physiology Learning System, 2nd ed. Philadelphia, W. B. Saunders Company, 2000.)

meningitis *(continued)*
    basilar m.
    benign lymphocytic m.
    m. carcinomatosa
    carcinomatous m.
    cerebral m.
    cerebrospinal m.
    chronic m.
    cryptococcal m.
    eosinophilic m.
    epidemic cerebrospinal m.
    external m.
    gummatous m.
    Haemophilus influenzae m.
    internal m.
    lymphocytic m.
    meningococcal m.
    Mollaret's m.
    mumps m.
    neoplastic m.
    occlusive m.
    m. ossificans
    otitic m.
    pneumococcal m.
    purulent m.
    pyogenic m.
    m. serosa circumscripta
    spinal m.
    sterile m.
    m. sympathica
    syphilitic m.
    tubercular m.
    tuberculous m.
    viral m.

meningoarteritis

meningocele
    anterior m.
    cranial m.
    sacral m.
    spinal m.
    spurious m.
    traumatic m.

meningocephalitis

meningocerebritis

meningococcemia
    acute fulminating m.

meningocortical

meningocyte

meningoencephalitis
    amebic m.
    eosinophilic m.
    mumps m.
    primary amebic m.
    syphilitic m.
    toxoplasmic m.

meningoencephalocele

meningoencephalomyelitis

meningoencephalomyelopathy

meningoencephalopathy

meningofibroblastoma

meningogenic

meningoma

meningomyelitis
    syphilitic m.

meningomyelocele

meningomyeloencephalitis

meningomyeloradiculitis

meningopathy

meningopolyneuritis

meningorachidian

meningoradicular

meningoradiculitis

meningorrhagia

meningorrhea

meningothelioma

meningovascular

meninx *(singular of* meninges)

meniscus *pl.* menisci
    m. tactus

Menkes' kinky-hair syndrome

mental age

Menzel's ataxia

meralgia
    m. paresthetica

Meretoja
    M's syndrome
    M. type familial amyloid
      polyneuropathy

Merkel
    M. cell
    M's corpuscle
    M's disk
    M. tactile cell

merlin

merocoxalgia

merorachischisis

merosmia

MERRF syndrome

Merzbacher-Pelizaeus disease

mesaxon

mesencephalic

mesencephalitis

mesencephalohypophyseal

mesencephalon

mesencephalotomy

mesocortex

Mestinon

metatarsalgia
    Morton's m.

metathalamus

metatherian

metencephalic

metencephalon

metencephalospinal

met-enkephalin

method
    Kety-Schmidt m.

method *(continued)*
    Thane's m.

N-methyl-D-aspartate

metonymy

Meyer
    M's loop
    M.-Archambault loop

Meynert
    basal nucleus of M.
    M's bundle
    M's cells
    M's commissure
    M's fasciculus
    fountain decussation of M.
    M's layer
    M's nucleus
    nucleus basalis of M.
    solitary cells of M.
    M's tract

mication

microcyte

microdysgenesia

microglia

microgliacyte

microglial

microgliocyte

microglioma

microgliomatosis

micrographia

microgyrus

microneurography

microneurosurgery

micropituicyte

micropsia

microptic

midbrain

midface hypoplasia syndrome

midtegmentum

Mierzejewski effect

migraine
    m. accompagnée
    abdominal m.
    m. with aura
    m. without aura
    acute confusional m.
    basilar m.
    basilar artery m.
    Bickerstaff's m.
    cardiac m.
    cervical m.
    classic m.
    common m.
    complicated m.
    dysphrenic m.
    familial hemiplegic m.
    hemiplegic m.
    m. sans m.
    neurologic m.
    ocular m.
    ophthalmoplegic m.
    ophthalmic m.
    m. psychosis
    retinal m.

migraineur

migrainoid

migrainous

milk
    uterine m.

Millard
    M.-Gubler paralysis
    M.-Gubler syndrome

Miller Fisher syndrome

Miller-Dieker syndrome

minimum
    m. sensibile
    m. separabile

Minnesota Multiphasic Personality Inventory (MMPI)

Minor
    M's disease
    M's sign

Mirapex

miryachit

MMPI
    Minnesota Multiphasic Personality Inventory

Möbius
    M's disease
    M's syndrome

modality

Monakow
    M's bundle
    M's fasciculus
    fasciculus aberrans of M.
    M's fibers
    M's nucleus
    M's syndrome
    M's tract

monathetosis

Mondini syndrome

Mondonesi's reflex

monesthetic

monoaminergic

monochorea

monoganglial

monomyoplegia

mononeural

mononeuric

mononeuritis
    m. multiplex

mononeuropathy
    cranial m.
    m. multiplex
    multifocal m.
    multiple m.

monoparesis

monoparesthesia

monoplegia

monoplegic

monospasm

monosynaptic

Monro
    fissure of M.
    foramen of M.
    sulcus of M.
    M.-Kel Roussy-Lévy heredi-
        tary areflexic dystasia

montage

monticulus *pl.* monticuli
    m. cerebelli

Moore's syndrome

Morand's spur

Morgagni's tubercle

Morley's peritoneocutaneous
    reflex

Morton
    M's disease
    M's foot
    M's metatarsalgia
    M's neuralgia
    M's toe

Morvan's syndrome

motoceptor

motoneuron
    alpha m's
    beta m's
    gamma m's
    heteronymous m's
    homonymous m's
    lower m's
    peripheral m.
    upper m's

motor

motoricity

Mount
    M's syndrome
    M.-Reback syndrome

mouth
    tapir m.

movement
    associated m.
    athetoid m.
    automatic m.
    ballistic m's
    choreic m's
    choreiform m's
    circus m.
    contralateral associated m.
    dystonic m.
    forced m.
    involuntary m.
    Magnan's m.
    rapid eye m.
    reflex m.
    spontaneous m.
    synkinetic m.

MRI
    magnetic resonance imag-
        ing
        functional MRI
        perfusion MRI

MRS
    magnetic resonance spec-
        troscopy

Müller
    ganglion of M.

multicore disease

multielectrode

multiganglionic

multimodal

multiplet

multisensory

multisynaptic

mumps
    m. meningoencephalitis

Murray Valley
    M. V. disease
    M. V. encephalitis

muscarine

muscarinic

musicogenic

muscle
    homonymous m.

mussitation

mutism
    akinetic m.

myalgia
    m. capitis

myasthenia
    m. gravis
    m. gravis, familial infantile
    m. gravis pseudoparalytica

myasthenic

myatonia

myatony

myelalgia

myelapoplexy

myelatelia

myelatrophy

myelauxe

myelencephalitis

myelencephalon

myelin
    m. sheath

myelinated

myelination

myelinic

myelinization

myelinoclasis
    acute perivascular m.
    postinfection periven-
        ous m.

myelinogenesis

myelinogenetic

myelinogeny

myelinolysis
    central pontine m.

myelinopathy

myelinotoxic

myelinotoxicity

myelitic

myelitis
    acute m.
    ascending m.
    bulbar m.
    cavitary m.
    central m.
    chronic m.
    compression m.
    concussion m.
    cornual m.
    diffuse m.
    disseminated m.
    hemorrhagic m.
    neuro-optic m.
    periependymal m.
    postinfectious m.
    postvaccinal m.
    subacute m.
    subacute necrotic m.
    syphilitic m.
    transverse m.
    m. vaccinia
    viral m.

myeloarchitecture

myelocele

myeloclast

myelocystocele

myelocystomeningocele

myelodysplasia

myelodysplastic

myeloencephalic

myeloencephalitis
    eosinophilic m.

myeloencephalopathy

myelofugal

myelogenesis

myelogenic

myelogenous

myelogeny

myeloid

myelolysis

myelolytic

myelomalacia

myelomenia

myelomeningitis

myelomeningocele

myeloneuritis

myelo-opticoneuropathy
  subacute m.

myelopathic

myelopathy
  angiodysgenetic necro-
    tizing m.
  anterior m.
  ascending m.
  carcinomatous m.
  cervical spondylotic m.
  chronic progressive m.
  compression m.
  concussion m.
  cystic m.
  descending m.
  focal m.
  funicular m.
  hemorrhagic m.
  HTLV-1–associated m.
  necrotizing m.
  paracarcinomatous m.
  paraneoplastic m.
  radiation m.
  spondylotic cervical m.
  systemic m.
  transverse m.
  traumatic m.

myelopathy *(continued)*
  vacuolar m.

myelopetal

myelophthisic

myelophthisis

myeloplegia

myelopore

myeloradiculitis

myeloradiculodysplasia

myeloradiculopathy

myelorrhagia

myeloschisis

myelosclerosis

myelosis

myelosyphilis

myelotome

myelotomy
  Bischof's m.
  commissural m.

Myerson's sign

myesthesia

myobradia

myoclonia
  m. epileptica
  m. fibrillaris multiplex
  fibrillary m.

myoclonic

myoclonus
  action m.
  Baltic m.
  cortical m.
  cortical reflex m.
  epileptic m.
  essential m.
  intention m.
  m. multiplex
  nocturnal m.
  opsoclonus-m.

myoclonus *(continued)*
    palatal m.
    reflex m.

myocomma

myodystonia

myodystony

myodystrophia

myodystrophy

myohypertrophia
    m. kymoparalytica

myokymia

myoneural

myopalmus

myoparalysis

myoparesis

myopathy
    distal m.
    glycolytic m.
    late distal hereditary m.

myopathy *(continued)*
    lipid m.
    mitochondrial m.
    Welander's m.
    Welander's distal m.

myoschwannoma

myospasm

myospasmia

myotactic

myotonia
    m. congenita
    m. hereditaria
    m. tarda

myotonic

myotonoid

myotonus

myriachit

Mysoline

myxoglioma

Naffziger
  N's syndrome
  N's test

Nageotte
  N's bracelets
  N's cells

narcolepsy

narcoleptic

narcose

narcous

neck
  n. of dorsal horn of spinal
    cord
  n. of head of posterior
    horn of spinal cord
  n. of posterior horn of spi-
    nal cord

necrencephalus

neglect
  sensory n.
  unilateral n.
  hemispatial n.

Negri-Jacod syndrome

Negro
  N's phenomenon
  N's sign

Nélaton's syndrome

neocerebellum

neocinetic

neocortex

neoendorphin

neokinetic

neopallium

neostriatum

neothalamus

Neri's sign

nerve
  abducens n.

nerve *(continued)*
  abducent n.
  accelerator n's
  accessory n.
  accessory n., spinal
  accessory n., vagal
  acoustic n.
  afferent n.
  alveolar n., inferior
  alveolar n's, superior
  ampullar n., anterior
  ampullar n., inferior
  ampullar n., lateral
  ampullar n., posterior
  ampullar n., superior
  anal n's, inferior
  Andersch's n.
  anococcygeal n.
  antebrachial cutaneous n.,
    lateral
  antebrachial cutaneous n.,
    medial
  antebrachial cutaneous n.,
    posterior
  aortic n.
  Arnold's n.
  articular n.
  auditory n.
  auricular n's, anterior
  auricular n., great
  auricular n., internal
  auricular n., posterior
  auricular n. of vagus n.
  auriculotemporal n.
  autonomic n.
  axillary n.
  Bell's n.
  Bock's n.
  brachial cutaneous n., infe-
    rior lateral
  brachial cutaneous n., me-
    dial
  brachial cutaneous n., pos-
    terior
  brachial cutaneous n., su-
    perior lateral
  buccal n.
  buccinator n.

nerve *(continued)*
    cardiac n., inferior
    cardiac n., middle
    cardiac n., superior
    cardiac n's, supreme
    cardiac n's, thoracic
    caroticotympanic n's
    caroticotympanic n., inferior
    caroticotympanic n., superior
    carotid n's, external
    carotid n., internal
    cavernosal n's
    cavernous n's of clitoris
    cavernous n's of penis
    cavernous n. of penis, greater
    cavernous n's of penis, lesser
    celiac n's
    centrifugal n.
    centripetal n.
    cerebral n's
    cervical n's
    cervical n., descending
    cervical n., transverse
    cervical cardiac n., inferior
    cervical cardiac n., middle
    cervical cardiac n., superior
    chorda tympani n.
    ciliary n's, long
    ciliary n's, short
    circumflex n.
    cluneal n's, inferior
    cluneal n's, middle
    cluneal n's, superior
    coccygeal n.
    cochlear n.
    n. of Cotunnius
    cranial n's
    cranial n., eighth
    cranial n., eleventh
    cranial n., fifth
    cranial n., first
    cranial n., fourth
    cranial n., ninth
    cranial n., second

nerve *(continued)*
    cranial n., seventh
    cranial n., sixth
    cranial n., tenth
    cranial n., third
    cranial n., twelfth
    crural interosseous n.
    cubital n.
    cutaneous n.
    cutaneous n's, femoral
    cutaneous n. of abdomen, anterior
    cutaneous n. of arm, inferior lateral
    cutaneous n. of arm, medial
    cutaneous n. of arm, posterior
    cutaneous n. of arm, superior lateral
    cutaneous n. of calf, lateral
    cutaneous n. of calf, medial
    cutaneous n. of foot, intermediate dorsal
    cutaneous n. of foot, lateral dorsal
    cutaneous n. of foot, medial dorsal
    cutaneous n. of forearm, dorsal
    cutaneous n. of forearm, lateral
    cutaneous n. of forearm, medial
    cutaneous n. of forearm, posterior
    cutaneous n. of neck, anterior
    cutaneous n. of neck, transverse
    cutaneous n. of thigh, intermediate
    cutaneous n. of thigh, lateral
    cutaneous n. of thigh, medial
    cutaneous n. of thigh, posterior
    Cyon's n.

nerve *(continued)*
  dental n., inferior
  depressor n.
  diaphragmatic n.
  digastric n.
  digital n's, radial dorsal
  digital n's, ulnar dorsal
  digital n's of foot, dorsal
  digital n's of lateral plantar n., common plantar
  digital n's of lateral plantar n., proper plantar
  digital n's of lateral surface of great toe and of medial surface of second toe, dorsal
  digital n's of medial plantar n., common plantar
  digital n's of medial plantar n., proper plantar
  digital n's of median n., common palmar
  digital n's of median n., proper palmar
  digital n's of radial n., dorsal
  digital n's of ulnar n., collateral palmar
  digital n's of ulnar n., common palmar
  digital n's of ulnar n., dorsal
  digital n's of ulnar n., proper palmar
  dorsal n. of clitoris
  dorsal n. of penis
  dorsal n. of scapula
  dorsal scapular n.
  efferent n.
  eighth n.
  eleventh n.
  encephalic n's
  ethmoidal n., anterior
  ethmoidal n., posterior
  exciter n.
  excitor n.
  excitoreflex n.
  n. of external acoustic meatus

nerve *(continued)*
  facial n.
  facial n., temporal
  femoral n.
  femoral cutaneous n., intermediate
  femoral cutaneous n., lateral
  femoral cutaneous n., medial
  femoral cutaneous n., posterior
  fibular n., common
  fibular n., deep
  fibular n., superficial
  fifth n.
  first n.
  fourth n.
  frontal n.
  furcal n.
  fusimotor n's
  Galen's n.
  gangliated n.
  gastric n's
  genitofemoral n.
  glossopharyngeal n.
  gluteal n's
  gluteal n., inferior
  gluteal n's, middle
  gluteal n., superior
  gustatory n's
  hemorrhoidal n's, inferior
  Hering's n.
  hypogastric n.
  hypoglossal n.
  hypoglossal n., descending
  iliohypogastric n.
  ilioinguinal n.
  iliopubic n.
  infraoccipital n.
  infraorbital n.
  infratrochlear n.
  inhibitory n.
  intercostal n's
  intercostobrachial n's
  intermediary n.
  intermediate n.
  interosseous n. of forearm, anterior

nerve *(continued)*
    interosseous n. of forearm,
        posterior
    interosseous n. of leg
    ischiadic n.
    Jacobson's n.
    jugular n.
    labial n's, anterior
    labial n's, posterior
    lacrimal n.
    n's of Lancisi
    Langley's n's
    laryngeal n., external
    laryngeal n., inferior
    laryngeal n., internal
    laryngeal n., internal supe-
        rior
    laryngeal n., recurrent
    laryngeal n., superior
    Latarjet's n.
    n. to lateral pterygoid
    n. to levator ani
    lingual n.
    longitudinal n's of Lancisi
    Ludwig's n.
    lumbar n's
    lumboinguinal n.
    n. of Luschka
    mandibular n.
    masseteric n.
    maxillary n.
    n. to medial pterygoid
    median n.
    meningeal n.
    mental n.
    mixed n.
    n. of mixed fibers
    motor n.
    motor n. of tongue
    musculocutaneous n.
    musculocutaneous n. of
        foot
    musculocutaneous n. of leg
    musculospiral n.
    myelinated n.
    mylohyoid n.
    n. to mylohyoid
    nasociliary n.
    nasopalatine n.

nerve *(continued)*
    ninth n.
    obturator n.
    obturator n., accessory
    obturator n., internal
    n. to obturator internus
    n. to obturator internus
        and gemellus superior
    occipital n., greater
    occipital n., least
    occipital n., lesser
    occipital n., smaller
    occipital n., third
    oculomotor n.
    olfactory n.
    ophthalmic n.
    optic n.
    pain n.
    palatine n., anterior
    palatine n., greater
    palatine n's, lesser
    palatine n., medial
    palatine n., middle
    palatine n., posterior
    parasympathetic n.
    parotid n's
    n. to pectineus
    pectoral n., lateral
    pectoral n., medial
    perforating cutaneous n.
    perineal n's
    peripheral n.
    peroneal n., accessory
        deep
    peroneal n., common
    peroneal n., deep
    peroneal n., superficial
    petrosal n., deep
    petrosal n., greater
    petrosal n., greater superfi-
        cial
    petrosal n., lesser
    petrosal n., lesser superfi-
        cial
    pharyngeal n.
    phrenic n.
    phrenic n's, accessory
    phrenicoabdominal n's
    pilomotor n's

nerve *(continued)*
    piriform n.
    n. to piriformis
    plantar n., lateral
    plantar n., medial
    pneumogastric n.
    popliteal n., external
    popliteal n., internal
    popliteal n., lateral
    popliteal n., medial
    presacral n.
    pressor n.
    pterygoid n., external
    pterygoid n., internal
    pterygoid n., lateral
    pterygoid n., medial
    n. of pterygoid canal
    pterygopalatine n's
    pudendal n.
    n. to quadratus femoris
    n. to quadratus femoris
      and gemellus inferior
    radial n.
    radial n., deep
    radial n., superficial
    rectal n's, inferior
    recurrent n.
    recurrent n., ophthalmic
    saccular n.
    sacral n's
    saphenous n.
    n. to sartorius
    scapular n., dorsal
    Scarpa's n.
    sciatic n.
    sciatic n., small
    scrotal n's, anterior
    scrotal n's, posterior
    second n.
    secretomotor n.
    secretory n.
    sensory n.
    seventh n.
    sinus n.
    sinu-vertebral n.
    sixth n.
    somatic n's
    spermatic n., external
    sphenopalatine n's

nerve *(continued)*
    n. to sphincter ani
    spinal n's
    splanchnic n's
    splanchnic n., greater
    splanchnic n., inferior
    splanchnic n., lesser
    splanchnic n., least
    splanchnic n., lowest
    splanchnic n's, lumbar
    splanchnic n's, pelvic
    splanchnic n's, sacral
    stapedial n.
    stapedius n.
    n. to stapedius
    stylohyoid n.
    stylopharyngeal n.
    subclavian n.
    subcostal n.
    sublingual n.
    submaxillary n's
    suboccipital n.
    subscapular n's
    sudomotor n's
    supraclavicular n's
    supraclavicular n's, ante-
      rior
    supraclavicular n's, inter-
      mediate
    supraclavicular n's, lateral
    supraclavicular n's, medial
    supraclavicular n's, middle
    supraclavicular n's, poste-
      rior
    n. to subclavius
    supraorbital n.
    suprascapular n.
    supratrochlear n.
    sural n.
    sural cutaneous n., lateral
    sural cutaneous n., medial
    sympathetic n.
    temporal n., anterior deep
    temporal n's, deep
    temporal n., middle deep
    temporal n., posterior deep
    temporal n's, subcutaneous
    n. to tensor tympani
    n. to tensor veli palatini

nerve *(continued)*
   tenth n.
   tentorial n.
   terminal n.
   third n.
   thoracic n's
   thoracic n., long
   thoracic splanchnic n., greater
   thoracic splanchnic n., lesser
   thoracic splanchnic n., lowest
   thoracodorsal n.
   tibial n.
   Tiedemann's n.
   tonsillar n's
   transverse n. of neck
   trigeminal n.
   trochlear n.
   twelfth n.
   tympanic n.
   ulnar n.
   unmyelinated n.
   utricular n.
   utriculoampullary n.
   vaginal n's
   vagus n.
   Valentin's n.
   vascular n's
   vasoconstrictor n.
   vasodilator n.
   vasomotor n.
   vasosensory n.
   vertebral n.
   vestibular n.
   vestibulocochlear n.
   vidian n.
   vidian n., deep
   visceral n.
   n. of Willis
   Wrisberg's n.
   zygomatic n.
   zygomaticofacial n.
   zygomaticotemporal n.

nervi *(plural of* nervus)

nervimotility

nervimotion

nervimotor

nervimuscular

nervomuscular

nervous

nervus *pl.* nervi
   n. abducens
   n. accessorius
   n. acusticus
   n. alveolaris inferior
   nervi alveolares superiores
   n. ampullaris anterior
   n. ampullaris lateralis
   n. ampullaris posterior
   nervi anales inferiores
   n. anococcygeus
   n. articularis
   nervi auriculares anteriores
   n. auricularis magnus
   n. auricularis posterior
   n. auriculotemporalis
   n. autonomicus
   n. axillaris
   n. buccalis
   n. canalis pterygoidei
   n. cardiacus cervicalis inferior
   n. cardiacus cervicalis medius
   n. cardiacus cervicalis superior
   nervi cardiaci thoracici
   nervi caroticotympanici
   nervi carotici externi
   n. caroticus internus
   nervi cavernosi clitoridis
   nervi cavernosi penis
   nervi cervicales
   nervi ciliares breves
   nervi ciliares longi
   nervi clunium inferiores
   nervi clunium medii
   nervi clunium superiores
   n. coccygeus
   n. cochlearis
   nervi craniales
   n. cutaneus

nervus *(continued)*

n. cutaneus antebrachii lateralis

n. cutaneus antebrachii medialis

n. cutaneus antebrachii posterior

n. cutaneus brachii lateralis inferior

n. cutaneus brachii lateralis superior

n. cutaneus brachii medialis

n. cutaneus brachii posterior

n. cutaneus dorsalis intermedius

n. cutaneus dorsalis lateralis

n. cutaneus dorsalis medialis

n. cutaneus femoralis lateralis

n. cutaneus femoralis posterior

n. cutaneus perforans

n. cutaneus femoris lateralis

n. cutaneus femoris posterior

n. cutaneus surae lateralis

n. cutaneus surae medialis

nervi digitales dorsales hallucis lateralis et digiti secundi medialis

nervi digitales dorsales nervi radialis

nervi digitales dorsales nervi ulnaris

nervi digitales dorsales pedis

nervi digitales palmares communes nervi mediani

nervi digitales palmares communes nervi ulnaris

nervi digitales palmares proprii nervi mediani

nervi digitales palmares proprii nervi ulnaris

nervus *(continued)*

nervi digitales plantares communes nervi plantaris lateralis

nervi digitales plantares communes nervi plantaris medialis

nervi digitales plantares proprii nervi plantaris lateralis

nervi digitales plantares proprii nervi plantaris medialis

n. dorsalis clitoridis

n. dorsalis penis

n. dorsalis scapulae

nervi encephalici

nervi erigentes

n. ethmoidalis anterior

n. ethmoidalis posterior

n. facialis

n. femoralis

n. fibularis communis

n. fibularis profundus

n. fibularis superficialis

n. frontalis

n. genitofemoralis

n. glossopharyngeus

n. gluteus inferior

n. gluteus superior

n. hypogastricus

n. hypoglossus

n. iliohypogastricus

n. ilioinguinalis

n. iliopubicus

n. infraorbitalis

n. infratrochlearis

nervi intercostales

nervi intercostobrachiales

n. intermediofacialis

n. intermedius

n. interosseus antebrachii anterior

n. interosseus antebrachii posterior

n. interosseus cruris

n. ischiadicus

n. jugularis

nervi labiales anteriores

nervus *(continued)*
    nervi labiales posteriores
    n. lacrimalis
    n. laryngealis inferior
    n. laryngealis recurrens
    n. laryngealis superior
    n. laryngeus inferior
    n. laryngeus recurrens
    n. laryngeus superior
    n. lingualis
    nervi lumbales
    nervi lumbares
    n. lumboinguinalis
    n. mandibularis
    n. massetericus
    n. maxillaris
    n. meatus acustici externi
    n. medianus
    n. meningeus medius
    n. mentalis
    n. mixtus
    n. motorius
    n. musculi obturatorii interni
    n. musculi piriformis
    n. musculi quadrati femoris
    n. musculi tensoris tympani
    n. musculi tensoris veli palatini
    n. musculocutaneus
    n. mylohyoideus
    n. nasociliaris
    n. nasopalatinus
    n. nervorum
    n. obturatorius
    n. obturatorius accessorius
    n. obturatorius internus
    n. occipitalis major
    n. occipitalis minor
    n. occipitalis tertius
    n. octavus
    n. oculomotorius
    n. olfactorius
    n. ophthalmicus
    n. opticus
    nervi palatini
    n. palatinus major
    nervi palatini minores

nervus *(continued)*
    n. pectoralis lateralis
    n. pectoralis medialis
    nervi perineales
    n. peroneus communis
    n. peroneus profundus
    n. peroneus profundus accessorius
    n. peroneus superficialis
    n. petrosus major
    n. petrosus minor
    n. petrosus profundus
    n. pharyngeus
    n. phrenicus
    nervi phrenici accessorii
    n. piriformis
    n. plantaris lateralis
    n. plantaris medialis
    n. presacralis
    n. pterygoideus lateralis
    n. pterygoideus medialis
    nervi pterygopalatini
    n. pudendus
    n. quadratus femoris
    n. radialis
    nervi rectales inferiores
    n. saccularis
    nervi sacrales
    nervi sacrales et n. coccygeus
    n. saphenus
    n. sciaticus
    nervi scrotales anteriores
    nervi scrotales posteriores
    n. sensorius
    n. spermaticus externus
    nervi spinales
    n. spinosus
    n. splanchnicus imus
    nervi splanchnici lumbales
    nervi splanchnici lumbares
    n. splanchnicus major
    n. splanchnicus minor
    nervi splanchnici pelvici
    nervi splanchnici sacrales
    n. splanchnicus thoracicus imus
    n. splanchnicus thoracicus major

nervus *(continued)*
n. splanchnicus thoracicus minor
n. stapedius
n. statoacusticus
n. subclavius
n. subcostalis
n. sublingualis
n. suboccipitalis
nervi subscapulares
nervi supraclaviculares
nervi supraclaviculares intermedii
nervi supraclaviculares laterales
nervi supraclaviculares mediales
nervi supraclaviculares posteriores
n. supraorbitalis
n. suprascapularis
n. supratrochlearis
n. suralis
nervi temporales profundi
n. tensoris veli palatini
n. terminalis
nervi thoracici
n. thoracicus longus
n. thoracodorsalis
n. tibialis
n. transversus cervicalis
n. transversus colli
n. trigeminalis
n. trigeminus
n. trochlearis
n. tympanicus
n. ulnaris
n. utricularis
n. utriculoampullaris
nervi vaginales
n. vagus
nervi vasorum
n. vertebralis
n. vestibularis
n. vestibulocochlearis
n. visceralis
n. zygomaticus

network
neurofibrillar n.

Neuhauser syndrome

neuragmia

neural
n. muscular atrophy

neuralgia
cervicobrachial n.
cervico-occipital n.
cranial n.
n. facialis vera
geniculate n.
glossopharyngeal n.
Hunt's n.
idiopathic n.
intercostal n.
mammary n.
migrainous n.
Morton's n.
nasociliary n.
occipital n.
otic n.
peripheral n.
postherpetic n.
sciatic n.
Sluder's n.
sphenopalatine n.
stump n.
supraorbital n.
trifacial n.
trifocal n.
trigeminal n.
Vail's n.
vidian n.

neuralgic

neuralgiform

neuranagenesis

neurapraxia

neurarchy

neuraxial

neuraxis

neure

neurectasia

neurectomy

neurectopia

neurectopy

neurepithelial

neurepithelium

neurergic

neurexeresis

neuriatry

neurilemma

neurilemmal

neurilemmitis

neurilemmoma

neurilemoma
    acoustic n.

neurility

neurimotility

neurimotor

neurinoma
    acoustic n.
    acoustic n., bilateral

neuritic

neuritis
    alcoholic n.
    brachial n.
    fallopian n.
    Gombault's n.
    hypertrophic n., interstitial
    intraocular n.
    lead n.
    leprous n.
    n. migrans
    migrating n.
    multiple n.
    optic n.
    optic n., orbital
    optic n., postocular
    optic n., retrobulbar
    periaxial n.
    peripheral n.
    radiation n.

neuritis *(continued)*
    radicular n.
    retrobulbar n.
    n. saturnina
    sciatic n.
    segmental n.
    serum n.
    shoulder-girdle n.
    syphilitic n.
    toxic n.
    vestibular n.

neuroacanthocytosis

neuroallergy

neuroamebiasis

neuroanastomosis

neuroanatomy

neuroastrocytoma

neurobiologist

neurobiology

neurobiotaxis

neuroblast
    sympathetic n.

neuroblastoma

neuroborreliosis

neuroceptor

neurochemistry

neurocirculatory

neurocladism

neurocommunications

neurocutaneous

neurocysticercosis

neurocytology

neurocytoma

neurodegenerative

neurodendrite

neurodendron

neurodevelopmental

neurodynia

neuroeffector

neuroelectricity

neuroencephalomyelopathy
    optic n.

neuroendocrine

neuroendocrinology

neuroepithelial

neuroepithelioma

neuroepithelium

neurofiber
    afferent n's
    association n.
    autonomic n's
    commissural n.
    efferent n's
    postganglionic n's
    preganglionic n's
    projection n.
    somatic n's
    tangential n's
    visceral n's

neurofibra
    neurofibrae afferentes
    n. associationis
    neurofibrae autonomicae
    n. commissuralis
    neurofibrae efferentes
    neurofibrae postgangliona-
        res
    neurofibrae postganglioni-
        cae
    neurofibrae pregangliona-
        res
    neurofibrae preganglioni-
        cae
    n. projectionis
    neurofibrae somaticae
    neurofibrae tangentiales
    neurofibrae viscerales

neurofibril

neurofibrilla

neurofibrillar

neurofibroma
    cutaneous n.
    dermal n.
    plexiform n.
    solitary n.

neurofibromatosis
    n. 1
    n. 2
    bilateral acoustic n.
    central n.
    peripheral n.

neurofibromin

neurofibrosarcoma

neurofilament

neurogangliitis

neuroganglion

neurogenetic

neurogenetics

neurogenic
    n. bladder

neurogenous

neuroglia
    interfascicular n.
    peripheral n.

neuroglial

neurogliocyte

neurogliocytoma

neuroglioma
    n. ganglionare

neurogliomatosis

neurogliosis

neuroglycopenia

neurohistology

neurohormonal

neurohormone

neurohumor

neurohumoralism

neurohypophyseal

neurohypophysectomy

neurohypophysial

neurohypophysis

neuroimaging studies
  cranial ultrasound
  CT (computed tomography)
  diffusion-weighed imaging
  functional magnetic resonance imaging
  magnetic resonance spectroscopy
  magnetic source imaging
  MRI (magnetic resonance imaging)
      perfusion MRI
  MRS (magnetic resonance spectroscopy)
  PET (positron emission tomography)
  SPECT (single photon emission computed tomography)
  XeCT (xenon-computed tomography)

neuroimmunomodulatory

neurokeratin

neurokinin

neurolemma

neurolinguistics

neurologia

neurologic

neurologist

neurology
  clinical n.

neurolues

neurolymphomatosis

neurolysis
  alcohol n.
  chemical n.
  intramuscular n.
  intrathecal n.
  phenol n.
  trigeminal n.

neurolytic

neuroma
  acoustic n.
  amputation n.
  amyelinic n.
  n. cutis
  false n.
  ganglionar n.
  ganglionated n.
  ganglionic n.
  medullated n.
  Morton's n.
  multiple n.
  myelinic n.
  nevoid n.
  plexiform n.
  stump n.
  n. telangiectodes
  traumatic n.
  true n.
  Verneuil's n.

neuromalacia

neuromalakia

neuromatosis

neuromatous

neuromechanism

neuromediator

neuromeningeal

neuromere

neurometabolic

neurometrics

neuromodulation

neuromodulator

neuromotor

neuromuscular

neuromyal

neuromyasthenia

neuromyelitis
    n. optica

neuromyic

neuromyositis

neuromyotonia

neuron
    afferent n.
    bipolar n.
    central n.
    connector n.
    efferent n.
    fusimotor n's
    Golgi type I n's
    Golgi type II n's
    intercalary n.
    intercalated n.
    internuncial n.
    local circuit n.
    lower motor n.
    motor n.
    multiform n.
    multimodal n.
    multipolar n.
    multisensory n.
    peripheral sensory n.
    piriform n's
    polymorphic n.
    postganglionic n's
    postsynaptic n.
    preganglionic n's
    premotor n.
    presynaptic n.
    primary sensory n.
    projection n.
    pseudounipolar n.
    Purkinje n's
    pyramidal n.
    secondary sensory n.
    sensory n.
    spiny n.
    unipolar n.

neuronal
    n. antibody
        anti-Ri
        anti-Hu
        anti-Yo

neurone

neuronitis
    vestibular n.

neuronopathy

neuronophage

neuronophagia

neuronotropic

Neurontin

neuro-oncology

neuro-otology

neuropacemaker

neuropapillitis

neuropathic

neuropathogenesis

neuropathogenicity

neuropathology

neuropathy
    acrodystrophic n.
    alcoholic n.
    amyloid n.
    angiopathic n.
    arsenic n.
    arsenical n.
    ascending n.
    autonomic n.
    axonal n.
    brachial plexus n.
    compression n.
    Dejerine-Sottas n.
    Denny-Brown's sensory n.
    Denny-Brown's sensory
        radicular n.
    descending n.
    diabetic n.

neuropathy *(continued)*
    entrapment n.
    femoral n.
    giant axonal n.
    hepatic n.
    hypertrophic n., hereditary
    hypertrophic n., progres-
      sive
    hypertrophic interstitial n.
    ischemic n.
    isoniazid n.
    lead n.
    lumbar plexus n.
    lumbosacral plexus n.
    motor n.
    motor and sensory n., he-
      reditary
    multiple n.
    nitrofurantoin n.
    nutritional n.
    paraneoplastic n.
    periaxial n.
    peripheral n.
    porphyric n.
    pressure n.
    sacral plexus n.
    sarcoid n.
    segmental (demyelina-
      tion) n.
    senile n.
    sensorimotor n.
    sensory n.
    sensory n., hereditary
    sensory and autonomic n.,
      hereditary
    sensory and motor n., he-
      reditary
    sensory radicular n., hered-
      itary
    serum n.
    serum sickness n.
    suprascapular n.
    tomaculous n.
    toxic n.
    traumatic n.
    vasculitic n.
neuropeptide
    n. Y

neurophilic
neurophysiology
neuropil
neuropile
neuroplasm
neuroplasmic
neuroplasty
neuroplexus
neuropodion
neuropodium
neuroprotection
neuroprotective
neuropsychological
    n. testing
neuropsychology
neurorrhaphy
neurosarcocleisis
neurosarcoma
neuroscience
neuroscientist
neurosecretion
neurosecretory
neurosegmental
neurosensory
neuroskeletal
neurosome
neurospasm
neurosplanchnic
neurospongioma
neurostatus
neurostimulation
neurosurgeon

neurosurgery
  functional n.
  stereotactic n.

neurosuture

neurosyphilis
  asymptomatic n.
  meningovascular n.
  parenchymatous n.
  paretic n.
  tabetic n.

neurotendinous

neurotensin

neuroterminal

neurothele

neurotization

neurotmesis

neurotome

neurotomy
  radiofrequency n.
  retrogasserian n.

neurotony

neurotransducer

neurotransmission

neurotransmitter
  false n.

neurotrauma

neurotrophic

neurotrophin

neurotrophy

neurotropic

neurotropism

neurotropy

neurotrosis

neurotubule

neurovaricosis

neurovascular

neurovegetative

neurovirulence

neurovirulent

neurovisceral

neururgic

neutropism

nevoid

Nicolau's septineuritis

nidal

nidus *pl.* nidi
  n. avis

Niemann
  N's disease
  N.-Pick disease

nigra

nigral

nigropallidal

nigrostriatal

Nissl
  N. bodies
  N. degeneration
  N's granules
  N's substance

nociassociation

nociception

nociceptive

nociceptor
  C-fiber n.
  cutaneous n's
  mechanical n.
  polymodal n.

nocifensor

nociperception

node
 Babès' n's
 n's of Ranvier

nodule
 Babès' n's
 n. of cerebellum
 Lisch n's
 n. of vermis

nodulus *pl.* noduli
 n. cerebelli
 n. vermis

noise
 end-plate n.

nonmedullated

nonmyelinated

non-neuronal

nootropic

noradrenaline

noradrenergic

no-reflow

norepinephrine

Norman
 N.-Roberts syndrome
 N.-Wood syndrome

Norrie's disease

nortriptyline

notch
 cerebellar n., anterior
 cerebellar n., posterior
 jugular n. of occipital bone
 jugular n. of temporal bone
 Kernohan's n.
 preoccipital n.
 tentorial n.

notencephalocele

Nothnagel's syndrome

notochordoma

NREM
 non–rapid eye movement
 NREM sleep

nuclear

nucleus *pl.* nuclei
 abducens n.
 n. abducens
 n. of abducens nerve
 n. abducentis
 n. accessorius columnae anterioris medullae spinalis
 nuclei accessorii nervi oculomotorii
 accessory n. of anterior column of spinal cord
 accessory basal amygdaloid n.
 n. of accessory nerve
 accessory oculomotor nuclei
 accessory nuclei of oculomotor nerve
 accessory olivary n., dorsal
 accessory olivary n., medial
 accessory olivary n., posterior
 accessory n. of ventral column of spinal cord
 n. accumbens
 n. accumbens septi
 acoustic nuclei
 nuclei of acoustic nerve
 n. alae cinereae
 n. ambiguus
 n. amygdalae
 n. amygdalae centralis
 n. amygdalae corticalis
 n. amygdalae lateralis
 amygdaloid n.
 amygdaloid n., central
 amygdaloid n., cortical
 amygdaloid n., lateral
 amygdaloid n., medial

nucleus *(continued)*
    amygdaloid n.
    n. amygdalae corticalis
    n. amygdalae centralis
    n. amygdalae medialis
    n. ansae lenticularis
    n. of ansa lenticularis
    n. amygdalae medialis
    n. anterior hypothalami
    anterior medial n. of oculo-
      motor nerve
    anterior olfactory n.
    anterior nuclei of thalamus
    nuclei anteriores thalami
    n. anterodorsalis thalami
    n. anteroinferior thalami
    n. anterolateralis medullae
      spinalis
    anterolateral n. of spinal
      cord
    n. anteromedialis medullae
      spinalis
    n. anteromedialis nervi
      oculomotorii
    n. anteromedialis thalami
    anteromedial n. of spinal
      cord
    anteromedial n. of thala-
      mus
    n. anterosuperior thalami
    n. anteroventralis thalami
    arcuate n. of hypothalamus
    arcuate n. of medulla ob-
      longata
    n. arcuatus hypothalami
    n. arcuatus medullae ob-
      longatae
    nuclei areae H, H_1, H_2
    auditory nuclei
    large cell auditory n.
    nuclei of auditory nerve
    autonomic n.
    autonomic oculomotor nu-
      clei
    n. autonomicus
    amygdaloid n., basal
    n. basalis telencephali
    basal nuclei
    basal n. of telencephalon

nucleus *(continued)*
    nuclei basales
    n. basalis of Meynert
    basal n. of Meynert
    bed n. of stria terminalis
    Bekhterev's (Bech-
      terew's) n.
    Bechterew's n.
    Blumenau's n.
    n. of Burdach's column
    n. caeruleus
    n. campi dorsalis
    n. campi medialis
    nuclei campi perizonalis
    n. campi ventralis
    caudal n., central
    nuclei of caudal colliculus
    n. caudalis centralis
    central caudate n.
    n. caudatus
    central lateral n. of thala-
      mus
    central medial n. of thala-
      mus
    central n. of spinal cord
    n. centralis medullae spina-
      lis
    n. centralis medullae spina-
      lis
    n. centralis lateralis thal-
      ami
    n. centralis medialis thal-
      ami
    n. centralis superior raphes
    n. centromedianus thalami
    cerebellar n., lateral
    cerebellar n., medial
    nuclei cerebellares
    nuclei cerebelli
    n. ceruleus
    cervical n., lateral
    n. cervicalis lateralis
    Clarke's n.
    cochlear nuclei
    cochlear n., anterior
    cochlear n., dorsal
    cochlear n., posterior
    cochlear n., ventral
    nuclei of cochlear nerve

nucleus *(continued)*

nuclei cochleares
n. cochlearis anterior
n. cochlearis dorsalis
n. cochlearis posterior
n. cochlearis ventralis
n. coeruleus
nuclei colliculi caudalis
nuclei colliculi inferioris
n. commissuralis nervi vagi
n. commissuralis rhomboidalis
n. commissurae posterioris
n. corporis geniculati lateralis
nuclei corporis geniculati medialis
n. corporis mammillaris medialis/lateralis
n. of cranial nerve
cuneate n.
cuneate n., accessory
cuneate n., lateral
n. cuneatus
n. cuneatus accessorius
n. cuneiformis
n. cuneiformis mesencephalicus
Darkshevich's n.
Deiters' n.
dentate n.
dentate n. of cerebellum
n. dentatus
dorsal n. of Clarke
dorsal column nuclei
n. of dorsal field
n. dorsalis corporis geniculati lateralis
n. dorsalis corporis geniculati medialis
n. dorsalis hypothalami
n. dorsalis lateralis thalami
n. dorsalis nervi oculomotorii
n. dorsalis nervi vagi
n. dorsalis raphes
nuclei dorsales thalami
dorsal lateral n. of thalamus

nucleus *(continued)*

dorsal n. of medial geniculate body
dorsal medial n. of thalamus
dorsal n. of oculomotor nerve
dorsal raphe n.
dorsal nuclei of thalamus
dorsal n. of vagus nerve
dorsolateral n. of oculomotor nuclear complex
dorsolateral n. of spinal cord
dorsomedial n. of intermediate hypothalamus
dorsomedial n. of thalamus
dorsomedial n. of spinal cord
n. dorsomedialis hypothalamicae intermediae
n. dorsomedialis medullae spinalis
Edinger's nuclei
Edinger-Westphal nuclei
n. emboliformis
n. endopeduncularis
entopeduncular n.
n. entopeduncularis
n. dorsolateralis medullae spinalis
n. of facial nerve
n. facialis
fastigial n.
n. fastigiatus
n. fastigii
nuclei formationis reticularis trunco encephalico
n. gelatinosus
geniculate n., dorsal lateral
geniculate n., lateral
geniculate nuclei, medial
geniculate n., ventral lateral
n. geniculatus lateralis
nuclei geniculati mediales
gigantocellular n.
n. globosus
n. gigantocellularis

nucleus *(continued)*

    n. of glossopharyngeal
        nerve
    n. of Goll's column
    n. gracilis
    nuclei of habenula
    nuclei habenulae
    habenular n., lateral
    habenular n., medial
    n. habenularis lateralis
    n. habenularis medialis
    hypoglossal n.
    n. hypoglossalis
    n. of hypoglossal nerve
    hypothalamic n., anterior
    hypothalamic n., dorsal
    hypothalamic n., dorsome-
        dial
    hypothalamic n., posterior
    hypothalamic n., ventrolat-
        eral
    hypothalamic n., ventrome-
        dial
    n. hypothalamicus anterior
    n. hypothalamicus dorsalis
    n. hypothalamicus dorso-
        medialis
    n. hypothalamicus poste-
        rior
    n. hypothalamicus ventro-
        lateralis
    n. hypothalamicus ventro-
        medialis
    nuclei of inferior colliculus
    inferior n. of trigeminal
        nerve
    n. inferior nervi trigemin-
        alis
    infundibular n.
    n. infundibularis
    n. intercalatus
    n. intermediolateralis me-
        dullae spinalis
    n. intermediomedialis me-
        dullae spinalis
    n. interpeduncularis
    interposed n., anterior
    interposed n., posterior
    n. interpositus anterior

nucleus *(continued)*

    n. interpositus posterior
    n. interstitialis
    interstitial n. of Cajal
    intracerebellar nuclei
    intralaminar nuclei of thala-
        mus
    nuclei intralaminares thal-
        ami
    Kölliker-Fuse n.
    lateral dorsal n. of thala-
        mus
    n. of lateral geniculate
        body
    n. lateralis cerebelli
    n. lateralis dorsalis thalami
    n. lateralis posterior thal-
        ami
    nuclei of lateral lemniscus
    lateral n. of mammillary
        body
    n. of lateral olfactory stria
    lateral posterior n. of thala-
        mus
    lateral ventral nuclei of
        thalamus
    nuclei lemnisci lateralis
    lenticular n.
    n. lenticularis
    n. lentiformis
    linear n., inferior
    linear n., intermediate
    linear n., superior
    n. linearis inferioris
    n. linearis intermedius
    n. linearis superior
    n. of Luys
    magnus raphe n.
    n. mammillaris lateralis
    n. mammillaris medialis
    masticatory n.
    medial central n. of thala-
        mus
    medial dorsal n. of thala-
        mus
    n. medialis cerebelli
    n. medialis magnocellularis
        corporis geniculati
    n. medialis dorsalis thalami

nucleus *(continued)*

    nuclei mediales thalami
    medial magnocellular n. of
      medial geniculate body
    medial n. of mammillary
      body
    n. of medial field
    nuclei of medial geniculate
      body
    medial nuclei of thalamus
    median raphe n.
    median nuclei of thalamus
    nuclei mediani thalami me-
      dialis
    n. mediodorsalis thalami
    mesencephalic trigemin-
      al n.
    mesencephalic n. of trigem-
      inal nerve
    n. of mesencephalic tract
      of trigeminal nerve
    n. mesencephalicus nervi
      trigemini
    n. mesencephalicus trige-
      minalis
    Meynert's n.
    midline nuclei of thalamus
    Monakow's n.
    motor n.
    motor n. of facial nerve
    n. motorius nervi trigemini
    n. motorius trigeminalis
    n. nervi abducentis
    n. nervi accessorii
    nuclei nervi cochlearis
    n. nervi cranialis
    n. nervi facialis
    n. nervi glossopharyngei
    n. nervi hypoglossi
    n. nervi oculomotorii
    n. nervi phrenici
    n. nervi pudendi
    nuclei nervi trigeminalis
    nuclei nervi trigemini
    n. nervi trochlearis
    nuclei nervi vagi
    nuclei nervi vestibulococh-
      learis
    obscurus raphe n.

nucleus *(continued)*

    n. obscurus
    oculomotor n. raphes
    n. oculomotorius
    nuclei oculomotorii acces-
      sorii
    nuclei oculomotorii auton-
      omici
    n. of oculomotor nerve
    n. olfactorius anterior
    n. olivaris accessorius dor-
      salis
    n. olivaris accessorius me-
      dialis
    n. olivaris accessorius pos-
      terior
    nuclei olivares caudales
    n. olivaris cranialis
    nuclei olivares inferiores
    n. olivaris rostralis
    n. olivaris superior
    olivary n.
    olivary nuclei, caudal
    olivary n., cranial
    olivary n., dorsal accessory
    olivary nuclei, inferior
    olivary n., posterior acces-
      sory
    olivary n., rostral
    olivary n., superior
    Onuf's n.
    n. of Onufrowicz
    n. originis
    pallidal raphe n.
    n. pallidus raphes
    parabrachial nuclei
    parabrachial n., lateral
    parabrachial n., medial
    nuclei parabrachiales
    n. parabrachialis lateralis
    n. parabrachialis medialis
    n. paracentralis thalami
    n. parafascicularis thalami
    paragigantocellular n., lat-
      eral
    n. paragigantocellularis lat-
      eralis
    paramedian n., dorsal
    paramedian n., posterior

nucleus *(continued)*
    n. paramedianus dorsalis
    n. paramedianus posterior
    n. parasolitarius
    nuclei parasympathici sacrales
    n. parataenialis thalami
    paratenial n. of thalamus
    paraventricular n. of hypothalamus
    n. paraventricularis hypothalami
    n. paraventricularis anterior thalami
    n. paraventricularis posterior thalami
    nuclei paraventriculares thalami
    paraventricular nuclei of thalamus
    paraventricular n. of thalamus, anterior
    paraventricular n. of thalamus, posterior
    pedunculopontine tegmental n.
    perihypoglossal nuclei
    nuclei perihypoglossales
    n. periventricularis posterior
    nuclei of perizonal field
    Perlia's n.
    phrenic n.
    phrenic n. of anterior column of spinal cord
    n. of phrenic nerve
    n. phrenicus columnae anterioris medullae spinalis
    nuclei of pons
    nuclei pontis
    n. pontis raphes
    pontine nuclei
    pontine raphe n.
    pontine n. of raphe
    pontine n. of trigeminal nerve
    pontine reticular n., caudal
    pontine reticular n., inferior intermediate

nucleus *(continued)*
    pontine reticular nuclei, intermediate
    pontine reticular n., oral
    pontine reticular n., superior intermediate
    pontine reticular n., tegmental
    n. pontinus nervi trigeminalis
    n. of posterior commissure
    n. posterior hypothalami
    posterior n. of hypothalamus
    n. posterior nervi vagi
    posterior n. of oculomotor nerve
    posterior raphe n.
    n. posterior raphes
    posterior periventricular n.
    posterior nuclei of thalamus
    nuclei posteriores thalami
    posterior n. of vagus nerve
    n. posterolateralis medullae spinalis
    n. posteromedialis medullae spinalis
    pregeniculate n.
    n. pregeniculatus
    preoptic n., lateral
    preoptic n., medial
    preoptic n., median
    preoptic n., periventricular
    n. preopticus lateralis
    n. preopticus medialis
    n. preopticus medianus
    n. preopticus periventricularis
    n. prepositus
    n. of prerubral field
    nuclei pretectales
    n. principalis nervi trigemini
    principal sensory n. of trigeminal nerve
    n. proprius
    n. of pudendal nerve
    n. pulposus, herniated

nucleus *(continued)*

    n. pulposus disci interver-
tebralis

    n. pulposus

    pulpy n. of intervertebral
disk

    nuclei pulvinares thalami

    raphe nuclei

    nuclei of raphe

    nuclei raphes

    n. raphes dorsalis

    n. raphes magnus

    n. raphes medianus

    n. raphes obscurus

    n. raphes pallidus

    n. raphes pontis

    n. raphes posterior

    red n.

    reticular nuclei

    reticular n., caudal pontine

    n. reticularis pontis ros-
tralis

    reticular n., gigantocellular

    reticular n., gigantocellular
intermediate

    reticular n., lateral

    reticular nuclei, lateral col-
umn

    reticular n., magnocellular

    reticular nuclei, medial col-
umn

    reticular nuclei, median
column

    reticular n., oral pontine

    reticular n., paramedian

    reticular n., parvocellular

    reticular nuclei, pontine

    reticular n., tegmental pon-
tine

    reticular nuclei of brain
stem

    nuclei of the reticular for-
mation

    reticular n. of medulla ob-
longata, intermediate

    reticular n. of medulla ob-
longata, lateral

    reticular nuclei of raphe

    reticular n. of tegmentum

nucleus *(continued)*

    reticular n. of thalamus

    nuclei reticulares

    n. reticularis intermedius
gigantocellularis

    n. reticularis intermedius
medullae oblongatae

    n. reticularis intermedius
pontis inferioris

    n. reticularis intermedius
pontis superioris

    n. reticularis lateralis me-
dullae oblongatae

    n. reticularis magnocellu-
laris

    n. reticularis paramedianus

    n. reticularis paramedianus
precerebelli

    n. reticularis parvocellu-
laris

    n. reticularis pontis cau-
dalis

    n. reticularis pontis oralis

    nuclei reticulares raphes

    n. reticularis tegmentalis
pedunculopontinus

    n. reticularis tegmentalis
pontinus

    n. reticularis tegmenti pon-
tis

    n. reticularis thalami

    reticulate n. of thalamus

    n. reticulatus thalami

    reticulotegmental n.

    n. retroambiguus

    retrodorsal n. of spinal
cord

    n. retrodorsolateralis me-
dullae spinalis

    retrofacial n.

    n. retrofacialis

    n. retroposterolateralis me-
dullae spinalis

    retroposterolateral n. of
spinal cord

    n. reuniens

    rhomboid n.

    n. rhomboidalis

    Roller's n.

nucleus *(continued)*
    roof nuclei
    n. ruber
    sacral parasympathetic nuclei
    n. salivarius inferior
    n. salivarius superior
    salivary n., inferior
    salivary n., superior
    n. salivatorius inferior
    n. salivatorius superior
    salivatory n., caudal
    salivatory n., inferior
    salivatory n., rostral
    salivatory n., superior
    Schwalbe's n.
    Schwann's n.
    n. semilunaris
    n. sensorius inferior nervi trigeminalis
    n. sensorius principalis nervi trigeminalis
    sensory n.
    sensory n. of trigeminal nerve, inferior
    sensory n. of trigeminal nerve, lower
    sensory n. of trigeminal nerve, principal
    septal n., lateral
    septal n., medial
    n. septalis lateralis
    n. septalis medialis
    Siemerling's n.
    nuclei solitarii
    solitary nuclei
    nuclei of solitary tract
    spherical n.
    spinal n. of accessory nerve
    n. of spinal tract of trigeminal nerve
    spinal n. of trigeminal nerve
    n. spinalis nervi accessorii
    n. spinalis nervi trigemini
    Spitzka's n.
    Staderini's n.
    Stilling's n.

nucleus *(continued)*
    striate n.
    n. striae terminalis
    n. subcaeruleus
    n. subceruleus
    n. subcuneiformis
    sublingual n.
    subparabrachial n.
    n. subparabrachialis
    n. subthalamicus
    superior central n.
    superior central raphe n.
    n. of superior olive
    suprachiasmatic n.
    n. suprachiasmaticus
    n. supraopticus
    n. tecti
    tegmental nuclei, anterior
    tegmental nuclei, ventral
    tegmental n., lateroposterior
    tegmental n., laterodorsal
    n. of tegmental field
    nuclei tegmentales anteriores
    n. tegmentalis posterolateralis
    n. tegmentalis pedunculopontinus
    tegmental pedunculopontine reticular n.
    nuclei tegmenti
    nuclei of tegmentum
    terminal n.
    n. terminationis
    thalamic nuclei
    thalamic nuclei, anterior
    thalamic nuclei, medial
    thalamic nuclei, median
    thalamic nuclei, posterior
    thalamic n., reticular
    thalamic nuclei, ventral
    nuclei of thalamus
    thoracic n.
    thoracic n., dorsal
    thoracic n., posterior
    n. thoracicus
    n. thoracicus dorsalis
    n. thoracicus posterior

nucleus *(continued)*

n. tractus mesencephalici nervi trigeminalis

nuclei tractus solitarii

nuclei of trapezoid body

triangular n.

n. triangularis

triangular septal n.

n. triangularis septi

trigeminal nuclei

trigeminal mesencephalic n.

trigeminal motor n.

nuclei of trigeminal nerve

trochlear n.

n. of trochlear nerve

n. trochlearis

nuclei tuberales laterales

vagal n., dorsal

n. vagalis dorsalis

nuclei of vagus nerve

ventral anterior n. of thalamus

n. of ventral field

ventral intermediate n. of thalamus

n. ventralis anterior thalami

n. ventralis corporis geniculati lateralis

n. ventralis corporis geniculati medialis

n. ventralis intermedius thalami

nuclei ventrales laterales thalami

nuclei ventrales mediales thalami

nuclei ventrales posteriores thalami

n. ventralis posterolateralis thalami

n. ventralis posteromedialis thalami

nuclei ventrales thalami

ventral lateral nuclei of thalamus

ventral medial n. of oculomotor nerve

nucleus *(continued)*

ventral medial nuclei of thalamus

ventral posterior nuclei of thalamus

ventral principal n. of medial geniculate body

ventral nuclei of thalamus

nuclei ventrobasales thalami

ventrolateral n. of hypothalamus

n. ventrolateralis hypothalami

n. ventrolateralis medullae spinalis

ventrolateral n. of spinal cord

ventrolateral nuclei of thalamus

nuclei ventrolaterales thalami

ventromedial n. of hypothalamus

n. ventromedialis hypothalami

n. ventromedialis medullae spinalis

ventromedial n. of oculomotor nuclear complex

ventromedial n. of spinal cord

vestibular n., caudal

vestibular n., cranial

vestibular n., inferior

vestibular n., lateral

vestibular n., medial

vestibular n., middle

vestibular n., rostral

vestibular n., superior

nuclei vestibulares

n. vestibularis caudalis

n. vestibularis inferior

n. vestibularis lateralis

n. vestibularis medialis

n. vestibularis rostralis

n. vestibularis superior

vestibulocochlear nuclei

nucleus *(continued)*
    nuclei of vestibulocochlear
      nerve
    Voit's n.
    Westphal's nuclei

numb

numbness

nutation

nutatory

nyctalgia

Nyssen-van Bogaert syndrome

nystagmus
    central n.
    convergence n.
    gaze n.
    gaze paretic n.
    palatal n.
    paretic n.
    resilient n.
    retraction n.
    n. retractorius
    rotary n.

nystagmus-myoclonus

obex

obliteration
cortical o.

oblongata

oblongatal

obnubilation

obtund

obtundation

obtundent

occipitothalamic

oculomotor
o. apraxia

oculospinal

odaxesmus

odaxetic

odogenesis

odor
minimal identifiable o.

odorant

odoriferous

odorimeter

odorimetry

odoriphore

odorivector

odorography

odynometer

oedipism

olfact

olfactant

olfaction

olfactism

olfactology

olfactometer

olfactometry

olfactory

olfactus

oligoastrocytoma

oligoblast

oligodendria

oligodendroblastoma

oligodendrocyte

oligodendroglia

oligodendroglioma

oligoglia

oligosynaptic

oliva

olivary

olive
accessory o's
inferior o.
superior o.

olivifugal

olivipetal

olivopontocerebellar

Ommaya reservoir

oneirophrenia

onomatopoeia

onomatopoiesis

Onuf's nucleus

Onufrowicz
nucleus of O.

Oort
bundle of O.

opalgia

operation
Cotte's o.
Dandy's o.

operation *(continued)*
   Frazier-Spiller o.
   Hartley-Krause o.
   Horsley's o.
   Körte-Ballance o.
   Krause's o.
   Torkildsen's o.

operculum *pl.* opercula
   frontal o.
   o. frontale
   frontoparietal o.
   o. frontoparietale
   opercula of insula
   occipital o.
   parietal o.
   o. parietale
   temporal o.
   o. temporale

ophthalmencephalon

ophthalmoneuritis

ophthalmoneuromyelitis

ophthalmoplegia
   o. plus

opioid

opisthion

opisthoporeia

opisthotonoid

opisthotonos

opisthotonus

opossum

Oppenheim
   O's reflex
   O's sign

opsialgia

opsoclonia

opsoclonus
   o.-myoclonus

opticochiasmatic

opticociliary

optochiasmic

Orap

organ
   Bidder's o.
   circumventricular o's
   effector o.
   end o.
   Golgi tendon o.
   gustatory o.
   lateral line o's
   neurotendinous o.
   olfactory o.
   parapineal o.
   parietal o.
   Ruffini's o.
   sense o's
   sensory o's
   o's of special sense
   subcommissural o.
   subfornical o.
   tendon o.
   terminal o.
   vascular o. of lamina terminalis

organoleptic

organum *pl.* organa
   o. gustatorium
   o. gustus
   o. olfactorium
   o. olfactus
   organa sensoria
   organa sensuum
   o. subcommissurale
   o. subfornicale
   o. vasculosum of lamina terminalis

orthochorea

orthodromic

orthotonos

orthotonus

os
   o. penis
   o. priapi

oscillopsia

Osler-Rendu-Weber syndrome

osmatic

osmesis

osmesthesia

osmics

osmoceptor

osmology

osmophore

osmoreceptor

osphresiology

osphresis

osphretic

ostium *pl.* ostia
    o. tympanicum tubae auditivae

otalgia
    geniculate o.

otalgia *(continued)*
    tabetic o.

Othello syndrome

otocerebritis

otoencephalitis

otoneurology

otorrhea
    cerebrospinal fluid o.

ototoxic

ototoxicity

overflow
    motor o.

overresponse

overventilation

ovoid
    myelin o's

oxcarbazepine

P

Pacchioni
    foramen of P.

pacchionian corpuscles

pachydermatocele

pachygyria

pachyleptomeningitis

pachymeninges

pachymeningitis
    cerebral p.
    circumscribed p.
    external p.
    hypertrophic cervical p.
    hypertrophic spinal p.
    internal p.
    p. intralamellaris
    purulent p.
    spinal p.
    syphilitic p.

pachymeningopathy

pachymeninx

Pacini's corpuscle

pacinian corpuscle

pain
    boring p.
    central p.
    fulgurant p's
    girdle p.
    heterotopic p.
    homotopic p.
    lancinating p.
    lightning p's
    phantom limb p.
    referred p.
    rest p.
    root p.
    shooting p's
    starting p's
    terebrant p.
    terebrating p.
    wandering p.

paleocerebellar

paleocerebellum

paleocortex

paleosensation

paleostriatal

paleostriatum

paleothalamus

palicinesia

palikinesia

palilalia

palingraphia

palinphrasia

paliphrasia

pallanesthesia

pallesthesia

pallesthetic

pallial

pallidal

pallidectomy

pallidoansection

pallidoansotomy

pallidofugal

pallidotomy

pallidum
    p. I
    p. II

Pallister-Hall syndrome

pallium

palpatometry

palsy
    Bell's p.
    brachial p.
    cerebral p.
    crossed leg p.
    Erb's p.

palsy *(continued)*
 Erb-Duchenne p.
 facial p.
 Klumpke's p.
 progressive bulbar p.
 progressive bulbar p. of
  childhood
 progressive infantile bulbar p.
 progressive supranu-
  clear p.
 pseudobulbar p.
 shaking p.
 spastic bulbar p.
 Saturday night p.
 tardy median p.
 tardy ulnar p.
 wasting p.

panautonomic

panencephalitis
 Pette-Döring p.
 subacute sclerosing p.

panesthesia

panesthetic

pang
 brow p.

panic attack

panodic

Pansch's fissure

pantalgia

panthodic

Papez circuit

papilla *pl.* papilli
 nerve p.
 nervous p.
 tactile p.

papilledema

papillitis

papilloma
 choroid plexus p.

para-analgesia

para-anesthesia

parabulia

paracerebellar

paracinesia

paracinesis

paraepilepsy

parafalx

paraflocculus
 ventral p.
 p. ventralis

parageusia

parageusic

paragraphia

parahippocampal

parakinesia

parakinetic

paralexia

paralexic

paralgesia

paralgesic

paralgia

paralogism

paralyses

paralysis
 acute ascending spinal p.
 p. agitans
 juvenile p. agitans
 alternate p.
 alternating p.
 ambiguo-accessorius p.
 ambiguo-accessorius-hy-
  poglossal p.
 ambiguospinothalamic p.
 juvenile p. agitans (of
  Hunt)
 ascending p.
 Avellis' p.

paralysis *(continued)*
- Bell's p.
- bilateral p.
- brachial p.
- brachial plexus p.
- brachial plexus p., lower
- brachial plexus p., upper
- brachiofacial p.
- Brown-Séquard's p.
- bulbar p.
- centrocapsular p.
- cerebral p.
- compression p.
- congenital abducens-facial p.
- congenital oculofacial p.
- crossed p.
- cruciate p.
- crural p.
- crutch p.
- Cruveilhier's p.
- decubitus p.
- Dejerine-Klumpke p.
- diaphragmatic p.
- Duchenne's p.
- Duchenne-Erb p.
- Erb's p.
- Erb-Duchenne p.
- facial p.
- false p.
- flaccid p.
- functional p.
- general p.
- glossolabial p.
- glossopharyngolabial p.
- Gubler's p.
- hereditary cerebrospinal p.
- hypoglossal p.
- infantile p.
- infantile cerebral ataxic p.
- infantile cerebrocerebellar diplegic p.
- infantile spinal p.
- Jamaica ginger p.
- juvenile p.
- Klumpke's p.
- Klumpke-Dejerine p.
- Kussmaul's p.
- Kussmaul-Landry p.

paralysis *(continued)*
- labial p.
- labioglossolaryngeal p.
- labioglossopharyngeal p.
- Landry's p.
- laryngeal p.
- lingual p.
- Lissauer's p.
- local p.
- masticatory p.
- medullary tegmental p's
- Millard-Gubler p.
- mimetic p.
- mixed p.
- motor p.
- musculospiral p.
- nuclear p.
- ocular p.
- oculomotor p.
- periodic p.
- peripheral p.
- peroneal p.
- phonetic p.
- postdormital p.
- postepileptic p.
- posthemiplegic p.
- posticus p.
- Pott's p.
- predormital p.
- pressure p.
- progressive bulbar p.
- pseudobulbar p.
- pseudohypertrophic muscular p.
- radial p.
- Ramsay Hunt p.
- reflex p.
- Remak's p.
- rucksack p.
- sensory p.
- sleep p.
- spastic p.
- spinal p.
- spinomuscular p.
- supranuclear p.
- tegmental mesencephalic p.
- Todd's p.
- trigeminal p.
- vasomotor p.

paralysis *(continued)*
    vocal cord p.
    vocal fold p.
    waking p.
    wasting p.

paralytic

paralytogenic

paralyzant

paralyze

paramnesia

paramusia

paramyoclonus
    p. multiplex

paramyotonia
    p. congenita

paranalgesia

paranesthesia

paraneural

paranomia

paranuclear

paraosmia

paraparesis
    spastic p. of the legs
    tropical spastic p.

paraphasia
    central p.
    literal p.

paraphasic

paraphemia

paraphia

paraphrasia

paraphrenia

paraphrenic

paraplectic

paraplegia
    alcoholic p.
    ataxic p.

paraplegia *(continued)*
    cerebral p.
    spastic p., congenital
    spastic p., Erb's
    spastic p., Erb's syphilitic
    flaccid p.
    spastic p., hereditary
    spastic p., infantile
    peripheral p.
    Pott's p.
    senile p.
    spastic p.
    spastic p., tropical
    p. superior
    syphilitic p.
    tetanoid p.
    toxic p.

paraplegic

paraplegiform

parapsia

parapsis

parareflexia

parasellar

parasomnia

parasympathetic

parasympathicotonia

parasympatholytic

parasympathomimetic

parathymia

paratonia

paraxon

parencephalocele

paresis
    general p.

paresthesia
    Bernhardt's p.

paresthetic

paretic

Parkes Weber syndrome

Parkinson
  P's disease
  P's facies
  P's mask
  P's sign

parkinsonian

parkinsonism
  postencephalitic p.

parolivary

parosmia

Parrot
  P's disease
  P's sign

Parry-Romberg syndrome

pars *pl.* partes
  p. abdominalis autonomica
  p. abdominalis systematis
    autonomici
  p. anterior commissurae
    anterioris
  p. anterior commissurae
    rostralis
  p. anterior lobuli quadran-
    gularis anterioris
  p. anterior pedunculi cere-
    bri
  p. anterior pontis
  p. autonomica systematis
    nervosi peripherici
  p. basilaris pontis
  p. basolateralis corporis
    amygdaloidei
  p. canalis nervi optici
  p. caudalis nervi vestibu-
    laris
  p. centralis systematis ner-
    vosi
  p. centralis ventriculi later-
    alis
  p. cervicalis medullae spi-
    nalis
  p. coccygea medullae spi-
    nalis
  p. cochlearis nervi octavi

pars *(continued)*
  p. cochlearis nervi vestibu-
    locochlearis
  p. compacta substantiae ni-
    grae
  p. corticomedialis corporis
    amygdaloidei
  p. cranialis partis parasym-
    pathici divisionis auton-
    omici systematis nervosi
  p. dorsalis corporis genicu-
    lati lateralis
  p. dorsalis corporis genicu-
    lati medialis
  p. dorsalis diencephali
  p. dorsalis lobuli quadran-
    gularis anterioris
  p. dorsalis pedunculi cere-
    bri
  p. dorsalis pontis
  p. duralis fili terminalis
  p. inferior nervi vestibu-
    laris
  p. inferoposterior lobuli
    quadrangularis
  p. infraclavicularis plexus
    brachialis
  p. intracanalicularis nervi
    optici
  p. intracranialis nervi op-
    tici
  p. intralaminaris nervi op-
    tici intraocularis
  p. intraocularis nervi optici
  p. lenticulothalamicus cap-
    sulae internae
  p. lumbalis medullae spina-
    lis
  p. lumbaris medullae spina-
    lis
  p. magnocellularis nuclei
    rubri
  p. nervosa neurohypophy-
    seos
  p. olfactoria corporis amyg-
    daloidei
  p. opercularis gyri frontalis
    inferioris

pars *(continued)*
    p. orbitalis gyri frontalis inferioris
    p. orbitalis nervi optici
    p. parasympathica divisionis autonomici systematis nervosi
    p. parvocellularis nuclei rubri
    p. pelvica autonomica
    p. pelvica partis parasympatheticae systematis nervosi autonomici
    p. pelvica systematis autonomici
    p. peripherica systematis nervosi
    p. pialis fili terminalis
    p. posterior commissurae anterioris
    p. posterior commissurae rostralis
    p. posterior lobuli quadrangularis anterioris
    p. posterior pedunculi cerebri
    p. posterior pontis
    p. postlaminaris nervi optici intraocularis
    p. prelaminaris nervi optici intraocularis
    p. reticularis substantiae nigrae
    p. retrolentiformis capsulae internae
    p. rostralis nervi vestibularis
    p. sacralis medullae spinalis
    p. spinalis nervi accessorii
    p. sublentiformis capsulae internae
    p. superior nervi vestibularis
    p. supraclavicularis plexus brachialis
    p. sympathica divisionis autonomici systematis nervosi

pars *(continued)*
    p. thalamolenticularis capsulae internae
    p. thoracica autonomica
    p. thoracica medullae spinalis
    p. thoracica systematis autonomici
    p. triangularis gyri frontalis inferioris
    p. vagalis nervi accessorii
    p. ventralis corporis geniculati lateralis
    p. ventralis corporis geniculati medialis
    p. ventralis diencephali
    p. ventralis lobuli quadrangularis anterioris
    p. ventralis pedunculi cerebri
    p. ventralis pontis
    p. vestibularis nervi octavi
    p. vestibularis nervi vestibulocochlearis

part
    abdominal autonomic p.
    abdominal p. of autonomic nervous system
    anterior p. of anterior commissure
    anterior p. of anterior quadrangular lobule
    anterior p. of cerebral peduncle
    anterior p. of pons
    autonomic p. of peripheral nervous system
    basilar p. of pons
    basolateral p. of amygdaloid body
    central p. of lateral ventricle
    cervical p. of spinal cord
    coccygeal p. of spinal cord
    compact p. of substantia nigra
    corticomedial p. of amygdaloid body

part *(continued)*

    cranial p. of parasympa-
thetic p. of autonomic division of nervous system

    craniosacral p. of auto-
nomic nervous system

    dorsal p. of anterior quad-
rangular lobule

    dorsal p. of lateral genicu-
late body

    dorsal p. of lateral genicu-
late nucleus

    dorsal p. of medial genicu-
late body

    dorsal p. of medial genicu-
late nucleus

    dural p. of filum terminale

    inferior p. of rhomboid
fossa

    inferior p. of vestibular
nerve

    infraclavicular p. of bra-
chial plexus

    intermediate p. of rhom-
boid fossa

    intracanalicular p. of optic
nerve

    intracranial p. of optic
nerve

    intralaminar p. of intraocu-
lar optic nerve

    intraocular p. of optic
nerve

    lumbar p. of autonomic
nervous system

    lumbar p. of spinal cord

    magnocellular p. of medial
geniculate body

    magnocellular p. of red nu-
cleus

    marginal p. of cingulate sul-
cus

    orbital p. of optic nerve

    parasympathetic p. of auto-
nomic division of nervous
system

    parvocellular p. of medial
geniculate body

part *(continued)*

    parvocellular p. of red nu-
cleus

    pelvic autonomic p.

    pelvic p. of autonomic ner-
vous system

    pelvic p. of parasympa-
thetic p. of autonomic division of nervous system

    pial p. of filum terminale

    posterior p. of anterior
commissure

    posterior p. of anterior
quadrangular lobule

    posterior p. of cerebral pe-
duncle

    posterior p. of pons

    postlaminar p. of intraocu-
lar optic nerve

    prelaminar p. of intraocular
optic nerve

    reticular p. of substantia ni-
gra

    retrolentiform p. of internal
capsule

    sacral p. of spinal cord

    spinal p. of accessory
nerve

    sublentiform p. of internal
capsule

    superior p. of rhomboid
fossa

    superior p. of vestibular
nerve

    supraclavicular p. of bra-
chial plexus

    sympathetic p. of auto-
nomic division of nervous
system

    thalamolenticular p. of in-
ternal capsule

    thoracic autonomic p.

    thoracic p. of autonomic
nervous system

    thoracic p. of spinal cord

    thoracolumbar p. of auto-
nomic nervous system

    vagal p. of accessory nerve

part *(continued)*
    ventral p. of anterior quad-
        rangular lobule
    ventral p. of cerebral pe-
        duncle
    ventral p. of lateral genicu-
        late body
    ventral p. of lateral genicu-
        late nucleus
    ventral p. of medial genicu-
        late body
    ventral p. of medial genicu-
        late nucleus
    ventral p. of pons

Patau's syndrome

path
    alvear p.

pathetic

pathway
    afferent p.
    auditory p.
    auditory p. central
    efferent p.
    final common p.
    gustatory p.
    internuncial p.
    motor p.
    olfactory p.
    perforant p.
    perforating p.
    sensory p.
    visual p.

pattern
    p. generator
    spike-and-wave p.

paucisynaptic

paw
    monkey p.

pectunculus

peduncle
    anterior p. of thalamus
    caudal p. of thalamus
    central p. of thalamus
    cerebellar p's
    cerebellar p., caudal

peduncle *(continued)*
    cerebellar p., cranial
    cerebellar p., inferior
    cerebellar p., middle
    cerebellar p., pontine
    cerebellar p., rostral
    cerebellar p., superior
    p's of cerebellum
    cerebral p.
    p. of cerebrum
    p. of flocculus
    inferior p. of thalamus
    p. of mammillary body
    olfactory p.
    pineal p.
    p. of pineal body
    posterior p. of thalamus
    superior p. of thalamus
    thalamic p's
    p's of thalamus

pedunculus
    pedunculi cerebellares
    p. cerebellaris caudalis
    p. cerebellaris inferior
    p. cerebellaris medius
    p. cerebellaris pontinus
    p. cerebellaris rostralis
    p. cerebellaris superior
    pedunculi cerebelli
    p. cerebralis
    p. cerebri
    p. corporis pinealis
    p. flocculi
    p. thalamicus inferior

Pelizaeus
    P.-Merzbacher disease
    P.-Merzbacher sclerosis

Pende's sign

Pendred's syndrome

penumbra
    ischemic p.

PEP syndrome

Pepper
    P. syndrome
    P. tumor

peptide
    calcitonin gene–related p.
    opioid p.

peptidergic

percept

perception
    stereognostic p.

perceptive

perceptivity

perceptorium

percipient

perencephaly

perfusion
    luxury p.

periaxonal

pericallosal

pericaryon

peridendritic

peridural

periencephalitis

periependymal

perigangliitis

periganglionic

periglial

peri-insular

perikarya

perikaryon

perimeningitis

perimyelitis

perineural

perineurial

perineuritic

perineuritis

perineurium

perinuclear

period
    absolute refractory p.
    latency p.
    latent p.
    refractory p.
    relative refractory p.

periostitis
    p. interna cranii

peripheraphose

peripherophose

perissodactylous

perisylvian

periventricular
    p. leukomalacia

Perroncito
    apparatus of P.
    P's spirals

perseveration

pes
    p. anserinus
    p. hippocampi
    p. pedunculi

petit mal

Pette-Döring panencephalitis

Pfeiffer syndrome

Phalen's maneuver

phantasm

phantogeusia

phantom

phantosmia

phase

phenobarbital

phenomenon
    arm p.
    Babinski's p.

phenomenon *(continued)*
- Bell's p.
- cheek p.
- clasp-knife p.
- cogwheel p.
- Cushing's p.
- Duckworth's p.
- Erben's p.
- face p.
- facialis p.
- finger p.
- Gowers' p.
- Grasset's p.
- Gunn's p.
- Grasset-Gaussel p.
- hip-flexion p.
- Hochsinger's p.
- Hoffmann's p.
- Holmes' p.
- Holmes-Stewart p.
- Hunt's paradoxical p.
- jaw-winking p.
- Kienböck's p.
- Leichtenstern's p.
- Lust's p.
- Marcus Gunn's p.
- Negro's p.
- no-reflow p.
- paradoxical diaphragm p.
- paradoxical p. of dystonia
- paradoxical pupillary p.
- peroneal nerve p.
- polyspike-spike wave p.
- Pool's p.
- Queckenstedt's p.
- radial p.
- rebound p.
- release p.
- Schlesinger's p.
- Schramm's p.
- Sherrington's p.
- Souques' p.
- springlike p.
- Strümpell's p.
- toe p.
- Trousseau's p.
- Wedensky's p.
- Westphal's p.

phenytoin

Philippe-Gombault
- tract of P.-G.
- triangular tract of P.-G.

Philippson's reflex

phlebitis
- sinus p.

phobia

phonomyoclonus

phose

phosis

photic stimulation

photoconvulsive

photoma

photomyoclonic

photomyogenic

photoparoxysmal

phrenemphraxis

phrenicectomy

phreniclasia, phreniclasis

phrenicoexairesis

phrenicoexeresis

phreniconeurectomy

phrenicotomy

phrenicotripsy

phrenoplegia

phrenospasm

physaliphore

pia

pia-arachnitis

pia-arachnoid

pia-glia

pia-intima

pial

pia mater
    p. m. cranialis
    p. m. encephali
    p. m. spinalis

piarachnitis

piarachnoid

Pick
    P. bodies
    P's disease

pickwickian syndrome

Pierre Robin syndrome

piesesthesia

piesimeter

piezesthesia

piezometer

pig

piitis

pillar
    anterior p. of fornix
    posterior p. of fornix

pill-rolling

pimozide

pineal

pinealectomy

pinealoblastoma

pinealocyte

pinealocytoma

pinealoma
    ectopic p.

pinealopathy

pineoblastoma

pineocytoma

Pierre Robin syndrome

Piotrowski's sign

Pitres' sign

pituicyte

pituitary
    posterior p.

pituitectomy

plaque
    argyrophil p's
    fibromyelinic p's
    p's jaunes
    Lichtheim p's
    neuritic p's
    Redlich-Fisher miliary p's
    senile p's

plasticity
    synaptic p.

plate
    end p.
    Kühne's terminal p's
    motor end p.
    quadrigeminal p.
    tectal p.
    terminal p.
    vascular foot p.

Plavix

pleocytosis

pleurothotonos

pleurothotonus

plexitis

plexopathy
    brachial p.
    lumbar p.
    lumbosacral p.
    sacral p.

plexus *pl.* plexus, plexuses
    p. of anterior cerebral artery
    aortic p., abdominal
    aortic p., thoracic
    p. aorticus abdominalis
    p. aorticus thoracalis
    p. aorticus thoracicus
    ascending pharyngeal p.
    Auerbach's p.

plexus *(continued)*
- auricular p., posterior
- p. autonomicus
- p. brachialis
- cardiac p.
- cardiac p., anterior
- cardiac p., deep
- cardiac p., great
- cardiac p., superficial
- p. cardiacus
- p. caroticus communis
- p. caroticus externus
- p. caroticus internus
- carotid p.
- carotid p., common
- carotid p., external
- carotid p., internal
- p. cavernosus
- cavernous p.
- celiac p.
- p. celiacus
- cervical p.
- cervical p., posterior
- p. cervicalis
- choroid p's
- choroid p., inferior
- p's of choroid artery
- choroid p. of fourth ventricle
- choroid p. of lateral ventricle
- choroid p. of third ventricle
- p. choroideus ventriculi lateralis
- p. choroideus ventriculi quarti
- p. choroideus ventriculi tertii
- p. coccygeus
- p. coeliacus
- colic p., left
- colic p., middle
- colic p., right
- coronary p's, gastric
- coronary p. of heart, anterior
- coronary p. of heart, left

plexus *(continued)*
- coronary p. of heart, posterior
- coronary p. of heart, right
- coronary p's of stomach, superior
- crural p.
- Cruveilhier's p.
- cystic p.
- p. deferentialis
- p. dentalis inferior
- p. dentalis superior
- diaphragmatic p.
- p. of ductus deferens
- p. entericus
- epigastric p.
- esophageal p.
- p. esophagealis
- p. esophageus
- Exner's p.
- external vertebral venous p.
- facial p.
- p. of facial artery
- p. femoralis
- gastric p's
- gastric p., inferior
- gastric p., left
- gastric p., superior
- p. gastrici
- gastroepiploic p., left
- hemorrhoidal p., middle
- hemorrhoidal p., superior
- p. hepaticus
- p. hypogasticus
- p. hypogastricus inferior
- p. hypogastricus superior
- ileocolic p.
- p. iliacus
- incisive p.
- infraorbital p.
- intermesenteric p., lumboaortic
- p. intermesentericus
- p. intraparotideus
- internal vertebral venous p.
- interradial p.
- intestinal p., submucous
- intramural p.

plexus *(continued)*
 ischiadic p.
 Jacobson's p.
 lienal p.
 p. lienalis
 lingual p.
 p. lumbalis
 p. lumbaris
 p. lumbosacralis
 maxillary p.
 maxillary p., external
 p. of medial cerebral artery
 Meissner's p.
 meningeal p.
 p. mesentericus inferior
 p. mesentericus superior
 molecular p.
 p. myentericus
 nasopalatine p.
 nerve p.
 p. nervorum spinalium
 nervous p.
 occipital p.
 p. oesophagealis
 p. oesophageus
 ophthalmic p.
 p. pancreaticus
 parotid p.
 p. parotideus
 patellar p.
 pelvic p.
 p. pelvicus
 p. pelvina
 p. periarterialis
 pharyngeal p.
 pharyngeal p., ascending
 p. pharyngealis nervi vagi
 pharyngeal p. of vagus
  nerve
 p. pharyngeus nervi vagi
 phrenic p.
 popliteal p.
 prevertebral p's
 prostatic p.
 p. prostaticus
 p. pulmonalis
 pulmonary p., anterior
 pulmonary p., posterior
 p. rectalis inferior

plexus *(continued)*
 p. rectalis medius
 p. rectalis superior
 p. renalis
 sacral p.
 p. sacralis
 Santorini's p.
 solar p.
 spermatic p.
 p. of spinal nerves
 p. splenicus
 p. subclavius
 submucosal p.
 p. submucosus
 subsartorial p.
 p. subserosus
 subtrapezius p.
 supraradial p.
 p. suprarenalis
 temporal p., superficial
 p. testicularis
 thyroid p., inferior
 thyroid p., superior
 tonsillar p.
 p. tympanicus
 p. tympanicus [Jacobsoni]
 p. uretericus
 uterine p.
 p. uterovaginalis
 vaginal p.
 vascular p.
 p. vascularis
 vertebral p.
 p. vertebralis
 vesical p.
 p. vesicale
 p. vesicalis
 vidian p.
 visceral p.
 p. visceralis

pli courbe

plumula

pneumatocele
 p. cranii
 extracranial p.
 intracranial p.

pneumatocephalus

pneumocephalus

pneumocrania

pneumocranium

pneumoencephalocele

pneumoencephalos

pneumorachis

pneumoventricle

pneumoventriculi

POEMS syndrome

point
Barker's p.
hysteroepileptogenous p.
hysterogenic p.
Keen's p.
Kocher's p.
motor p.
pressure p.
pressure-arresting p.
pressure-exciting p.
retromandibular tender p.
supraclavicular p.
supraorbital p.
vital p.
Vogt's p.
Vogt-Hueter p.
Ziemssen's motor p.

polarity
dynamic p.

pole
frontal p. of cerebral hemisphere
frontal p. of hemisphere of
cerebrum
occipital p. of cerebral
hemisphere
occipital p. of hemisphere
of cerebrum
temporal p. of cerebral
hemisphere
temporal p. of hemisphere
of cerebrum

poliencephalitis

poliencephalomyelitis

polio

poliodystrophia
p. cerebri
p. cerebri progressiva
p. cerebri progressiva in-
fantilis

poliodystrophy
progressive cerebral p.
progressive infantile p.

polioencephalitis
inferior p.

polioencephalomeningomyelitis

polioencephalomyelitis

polioencephalopathy

polioencephalotropic

poliomeningitis
nonparalytic p.

poliomyelencephalitis

poliomyelitis
abortive p.
acute anterior p.
acute lateral p.
anterior p.
ascending p.
bulbar p.
cerebral p.
endemic p.
epidemic p.
nonparalytic p.
paralytic p.
postinoculation p.
post-tonsillectomy p.
postvaccinal p.
spinal paralytic p.

poliomyeloencephalitis

poliomyelopathy

POLIP syndrome

pollodic

polus *pl.* poli
  p. frontalis hemispherii cerebri
  p. occipitalis hemispherii cerebri
  p. temporalis hemispherii cerebri

polyaxonic

polyesthesia

polyganglionic

polymyoclonus

polyneural

polyneuralgia

polyneuric

polyneuritic

polyneuritis
  acute febrile p.
  acute idiopathic p.
  acute infective p.
  acute postinfectious p.
  anemic p.
  cranial p.
  Guillain-Barré p.
  Jamaica ginger p.
  leprous p.
  postinfectious p.

polyneuromyositis

polyneuropathy
  acute postinfectious p.
  amyloid p.
  Andrade type familial amyloid p.
  anemic p.
  arsenic p.
  arsenical p.
  carcinomatous p.
  critical illness p.
  diphtheritic p.
  familial amyloid p.
  Finnish type familial amyloid p.
  idiopathic p.

polyneuropathy *(continued)*
  Indiana type familial amyloid p.
  inflammatory demyelinating p.
  Iowa type familial amyloid p.
  Japanese type familial amyloid p.
  Maryland type familial amyloid p.
  Meretoja type familial amyloid p.
  nutritional p.
  paraneoplastic p.
  porphyric p.
  Portuguese type familial amyloid p.
  Rukavina type familial amyloid p.
  symmetrical sensory p.
  uremic p.
  Van Allen type familial amyloid p.

polyneuroradiculitis

polypeptide
  vasoactive intestinal p.

polypeptidorrhachia

polyradiculitis

polyradiculoneuritis

polyradiculoneuropathy
  acute inflammatory demyelinating p.
  chronic inflammatory p.
  chronic inflammatory demyelinating p.
  chronic relapsing p.
  inflammatory demyelinating p.

polyradiculopathy

polysensitivity

polysensory

polysomnography

polyspike
  p.-spike wave phenomenon

polysynaptic

ponesiatrics

ponograph

pons
  p. cerebelli
  p. et cerebellum

pontes

pontile

pontine

pontobulbar

pontobulbia

pontocerebellar

pontocerebellum

pontomedullary

pontomesencephalic

pontopeduncular

Pool
  P's phenomenon
  P.-Schlesinger sign

pore
  gustatory p.
  taste p.

porencephalia

porencephalic

porencephalitis

porencephalous

porencephaly
  congenital p.
  encephaloclastic p.
  schizencephalic p.

porosis
  cerebral p.

Portuguese
  P. type familial amyloid
    polyneuropathy
  P.-Azorean disease

porus *pl.* pori
  p. gustatorius

position
  emprosthotonos p.
  opisthotonos p.
  orthotonos p.

postganglionic

postictal

postrolandic

postsylvian

postsynaptic
  p. neuron

posturing
  catatonic p.

potential
  acoustic evoked p.
  action p.
  after-p.
  auditory evoked p.
  bioelectric p.
  bizarre high-frequency p.
  brain stem auditory evoked
    p. (BAEP)
  compound action p.
  compound muscle action p.
  compound nerve action p.
  compound sensory nerve
    action p.
  cortical evoked p.
  demarcation p.
  electrical evoked p.
  end plate p.
  event-related p.
  evoked p.
  evoked cortical p.
  excitatory postsynaptic p.
    (EPSP)
  fasciculation p.
  fibrillation p.

potential *(continued)*
    generator p.
    inhibitory postsynaptic p.
    injury p.
    motor unit p.
    motor unit action p.
    muscle action p.
    myotonic p.
    negative after-p.
    nerve p.
    nerve action p.
    nerve fiber action p.
    positive after-p.
    postsynaptic p.
    readiness p.
    receptor p.
    resting p.
    resting membrane p.
    satellite p.
    sensory p.
    sensory nerve action p.
        (SNAP)
    serrated action p.
    somatosensory evoked p.
        (SSEP)
    spike p.
    visual evoked p. (VEP)
    visual evoked cortical p.

potentiation
    long-term p.
    posttetanic p.

Pott
    P's paralysis
    P's paraplegia

pouch
    Blake's p.

poverty
    p. of content
    p. of movement

Powassan encephalitis

PQ calcium channel

Prader-Willi syndrome

pragmatagnosia

pragmatamnesia

preataxic

precoma

precuneate

precuneus

prefrontal

pregabalin

preganglionic

preictal

preoptic

pressoreceptive

pressoreceptor

pressosensitive

pressure
    after p.
    cerebrospinal p.
    intracranial p.
    intrathecal p.

presubiculum

presylvian

presynaptic
    p. neuron

pretectal

pretectum

Prévost
    P's law
    P's sign

primary
    p. motor area

primate

primidone

prion

procedure
    activation p.
    Jannetta p.

process
    Deiters' p.
    dendritic p.

process *(continued)*
    p. of nerve cell
    p. of neuron
    sucker p.
    uncinate p.

processus
    p. intrajugularis ossis oc-
      cipitalis
    p. intrajugularis ossis tem-
      poralis
    p. jugularis ossis occipitalis

prodrome

proencephalon

Proetz test

progression
    backward p.
    cross-legged p.

projection
    eccentric p.
    thalamocortical p's

prolapse
    disk p.

proprioception

proprioceptive

proprioceptor

propriospinal

propulsion

prosencephalon

prosocele

prosocoele

prosopagnosia

prosopoplegia

Prostigmine test

protein
    encephalitogenic p.
    glial fibrillary acidic p.
    myelin basic p.
    myelin basic p. deficiency
    proteolipid p.

protein *(continued)*
    S-100 p.

protopathic

protrusion
    disk p.

proximoataxia

psalterial

psalterium

psammoma

psammomatous

pselaphesia

pseudagraphia

pseudaphia

pseudesthesia

pseudoagraphia

pseudoapoplexy

pseudoathetosis

pseudobulbar

pseudocele

pseudocephalocele

pseudoclonus

pseudocoele

pseudocoma

pseudodementia

pseudoesthesia

pseudoganglion
    Bochdalek's p.
    Cloquet's p.
    Valentin's p.

pseudographia

pseudomelia

pseudomeningitis

pseudomotor

pseudoneuroma

pseudoneuronophagia

pseudoparalysis

pseudopolycythemia
  paresthetic p.

pseudopolymelia

pseudosclerosis

pseudoseizure

pseudotabes
  diabetic p.
  pupillotonic p.

pseudotetanus

pseudotrismus

pseudotumor
  p. cerebri

pseudoventricle

pseudovertigo

psittacine

psychoacoustics

psychobiological

psychobiologist

psychobiology

psychomotor
  p. retardation

psychoneural

psychoneuroendocrinology

psychoses

psychosis
  acute delusional p.
  brief reactive p.
  functional p.
  migraine p.
  postpartum p.
  prison p.
  schizoaffective p.
  senile p.

psychosurgery

psychosurgical

psychotic

psychotropic

psychroalgia

psychroesthesia

ptosed

ptosis
  Horner's p.
  p. sympathetica

ptotic

puffer

puffer fish

pulp
  vertebral p.

pulse
  entoptic p.

pulvinar
  p. thalami

punchdrunk

punctum *pl.* puncta
  puncta vasculosa

puncture
  cisternal p.
  cranial p.
  intracisternal p.
  lumbar p.
  spinal p.
  suboccipital p.
  thecal p.
  ventricular p.

pupil
  Adie's p.
  fixed p.
  myotonic p.
  tonic p.

pupillatonia

pupillotonia

Purkinje
  P. cells
  P. cell layer

Purkinje *(continued)*
    P. layer
    P. neurons

purpura
    brain p.
    malignant p.

putamen

Putnam-Dana syndrome

Puusepp's reflex

pyencephalus

pyknoepilepsy

pyknomorphic

pyknomorphous

pyocephalus

pyramid
    p. of cerebellum
    Malacarne's p.
    p. of medulla oblongata
    p. of vermis

pyramidal

pyramidotomy

pyramis
    p. medullae oblongatae
    p. vermis
    p. bulbi

pyridoxine
    p.-deficiency seizure

quadriparesis

quadriplegia

Queckenstedt
    Q's phenomenon

Queckenstedt *(continued)*
    Q's sign
    Q's test

quisqualic acid

rachicentesis

rachiocentesis

rachiochysis

rachiomyelitis

rachischisis
    r. partialis
    r. posterior
    r. totalis

radiatio *pl.* radiationes
    r. acustica
    r. corporis callosi
    r. optica
    r. thalami anterior
    r. thalami centralis
    r. thalami inferior
    r. thalami posterior

radiation
    acoustic r.
    auditory r.
    r. of corpus callosum
    r. of Gratiolet
    occipitothalamic r.
    optic r.
    pyramidal r.
    tegmental r.
    thalamic r's
    thalamic r., anterior
    thalamic r., caudal
    thalamic r., central
    thalamic r., inferior
    thalamic r., posterior
    thalamic r., superior
    thalamostriate r.
    thalamotemporal r.
    r's of thalamus

radiationes (*plural of* radiatio)

radices (*plural of* radix)

radicotomy

radiculalgia

radicularis
    r. magna

radiculectomy

radiculitis

radiculoganglionitis

radiculomedullary

radiculomeningomyelitis

radiculomyelopathy

radiculoneuritis

radiculoneuropathy

radiculopathy
    cervical r.
    spondylotic caudal r.

radioencephalogram

radioencephalography

radioneuritis

radioreceptor

radiosurgery
    stereotactic r.
    stereotaxic r.

radix *pl.* radices
    r. anterior ansae cervicalis
    r. anterior nervi spinalis
    r. cochlearis nervi vestibu-
      locochlearis
    r. cranialis nervi accessorii
    r. dorsalis nervi spinalis
    r. facialis
    r. inferior ansae cervicalis
    r. inferior nervi vestibulo-
      cochlearis
    r. intermedia ganglii ptery-
      gopalatini
    r. lateralis nervi mediani
    r. lateralis tractus optici
    r. medialis nervi mediani
    r. medialis tractus optici
    r. motoria nervi spinalis
    r. motoria nervi trigemini

radix *(continued)*
  r. nasociliaris ganglii ciliaris
  r. oculomotoria ganglii ciliaris
  r. parasympathica ganglii ciliaris
  r. parasympathica ganglii otici
  r. parasympathica ganglii pterygopalatini
  r. parasympathica ganglii sublingualis
  r. parasympathica ganglii submandibularis
  r. parasympathica gangliorum pelvicorum
  radices plexus brachialis
  r. posterior ansae cervicalis
  r. posterior nervi spinalis
  r. sensoria ganglii ciliaris
  r. sensoria ganglii otici
  r. sensoria ganglii pterygopalatini
  r. sensoria ganglii submandibularis
  r. sensoria nervi spinalis
  r. sensoria nervi trigemini
  r. spinalis nervi accessorii
  r. superior ansae cervicalis
  r. superior nervi vestibulocochlearis
  r. sympathetica ganglii ciliaris
  r. sympathica ganglii ciliaris
  r. sympathica ganglii pterygopalatini
  r. ventralis nervi spinalis
  r. vestibularis nervi vestibulocochlearis

Radovici's sign

Raeder
  R's paratrigeminal syndrome
  R's syndrome

ramicotomy

ramisection

ramisectomy

Ramsay Hunt
  R. H. paralysis
  R. H. syndrome

ramus *pl.* rami
  r. albus nervi spinalis
  rami alveolares superiores anteriores nervi maxillaris
  r. alveolaris superior medius nervi maxillaris
  rami alveolares superiores posteriores nervi maxillaris
  r. anterior nervi auricularis magni
  rami anteriores nervorum cervicalium
  r. anterior nervi coccygei
  r. anterior nervi cutanei antebrachii medialis
  rami anteriores nervorum lumbalium
  r. anterior nervi obturatorii
  rami anteriores nervorum sacralium
  r. anterior nervi spinalis
  rami anteriores nervorum thoracicorum
  r. anterior sulci lateralis cerebri
  anterior rami of thoracic nerves
  r. articularis
  r. ascendens sulci lateralis cerebri
  r. auricularis nervi vagi
  r. autonomicus
  rami bronchiales anteriores nervi vagi
  rami bronchiales nervi vagi
  rami bronchiales posteriores nervi vagi
  rami buccales nervi facialis
  rami calcanei laterales nervi suralis

ramus *(continued)*

rami calcanei mediales nervi tibialis

rami cardiaci cervicales inferiores nervi vagi

rami cardiaci cervicales superiores nervi vagi

rami cardiaci thoracici

rami cardiaci thoracici nervi vagi

rami celiaci nervi vagi

r. cervicalis nervi facialis

rami clunium inferiores

rami clunium mediales

rami clunium superiores

rami coeliaci nervi vagi

r. colli nervi facialis

rami communicantes

r. communicans albus nervi spinalis

r. communicans cochlearis nervi vestibularis

r. communicans fibularis nervi fibularis communis

r. communicans griseus nervi spinalis

rami communicantes nervi auriculotemporalis cum nervo faciali

r. communicans nervi facialis cum nervo glossopharyngeo

r. communicans nervi glossopharyngei cum chorda tympani

r. communicans nervi glossopharyngei cum nervo auriculotemporali

r. communicans nervi glossopharyngei ramo meningeo nervi vagi

r. communicans nervi glossopharyngei cum ramo auriculari nervi vagi

r. communicans nervi intermedii cum nervo vago

r. communicans nervi intermedii cum plexu tympanico

ramus *(continued)*

r. communicans nervi lacrimalis cum nervo zygomatico

r. communicans nervi laryngei inferioris cum ramo laryngeo interno

r. communicans nervi laryngei superioris cum nervo laryngeo inferiore

r. communicans nervi lingualis cum chorda tympani

rami communicantes nervi lingualis cum nervo hypoglosso

r. communicans nervi mediani cum nervo ulnari

r. communicans cum nervo nasociliari

r. communicans nervi nasociliaris cum ganglio ciliari

rami communicantes nervorum spinalium

r. communicans nervi vagi cum nervo glossopharyngeo

r. communicans peroneus nervi peronei communis

r. communicans ulnaris nervi radialis

r. cutaneus

r. cutaneus anterior abdominalis nervi intercostalis

rami cutanei anteriores nervi femoralis

r. cutaneus anterior nervi iliohypogastrici

r. cutaneus anterior pectoralis nervi intercostalis

rami cutanei cruris mediales nervi sapheni

r. cutaneus lateralis abdominalis nervi intercostalis

r. cutaneus lateralis nervi iliohypogastrici

ramus *(continued)*

    r. cutaneus lateralis pecto-
       ralis nervi intercostalis

    r. cutaneus nervi obturato-
       rii

    r. cutaneus posterior rami
       posterioris nervi thoracici

    rami dentales inferiores
       plexus dentalis inferioris

    rami dentales superiores
       plexus dentalis superioris

    r. digastricus nervi facialis

    rami dorsales nervorum
       cervicalium

    r. dorsalis nervi coccygei

    rami dorsales nervorum
       lumbalium

    rami dorsales nervorum sa-
       cralium

    r. dorsalis nervi spinalis

    rami dorsales nervorum
       thoracicorum

    r. dorsalis nervi ulnaris

    rami esophagei nervi laryn-
       gei recurrentis

    r. externus nervi accessorii

    r. externus nervi laryngei
       superioris

    rami fauciales nervi lin-
       gualis

    r. femoralis nervi genitofe-
       moralis

    rami ganglionares nervi lin-
       gualis ad ganglion sub-
       mandibulare

    rami ganglionares nervi
       mandibularis ad ganglion
       oticum

    rami ganglionares nervi
       maxillaris ad ganglion
       pterygopalatinum

    rami gastrici anteriores
       trunci vagalis anterioris

    rami gastrici nervi vagi

    rami gastrici posteriores
       trunci vagalis posterioris

    r. genitalis nervi genitofe-
       moralis

ramus *(continued)*

    rami gingivales inferiores
       plexus dentalis inferioris

    rami gingivales nervi men-
       talis

    rami gingivales superiores
       plexus dentalis superioris

    rami glandulares ganglii
       submandibularis

    rami gluteales inferiores

    rami gluteales mediales

    rami gluteales superiores

    r. griseus nervi spinalis

    rami hepatici trunci vagalis
       anterioris

    r. inferior nervi oculomoto-
       rii

    rami inferiores nervi trans-
       versi colli

    r. infrapatellaris nervi sa-
       pheni

    rami interganglionares
       trunci sympathici

    r. internus nervi accessorii

    r. internus nervi laryngei
       superioris

    rami isthmi faucium nervi
       lingualis

    rami labiales nervi mentalis

    rami labiales superiores
       nervi infraorbitalis

    rami laryngopharyngei gan-
       glii cervicalis superioris

    r. lateralis nervi supraorbi-
       talis

    r. lateralis rami posterioris
       nervi cervicalis

    r. lateralis rami posterioris
       nervi lumbalis

    r. lateralis rami posterioris
       nervi sacralis

    r. lateralis rami posterioris
       nervi thoracici

    r. lingualis nervi facialis

    rami linguales nervi glosso-
       pharyngei

    rami linguales nervi hypo-
       glossi

ramus *(continued)*
 rami linguales nervi lingualis
 rami mammarii laterales
  rami cutanei lateralis pectoralis nervi intercostalis
 rami mammarii mediales
  rami cutanei anterioris pectoralis nervi intercostalis
 r. marginalis mandibularis nervi facialis
 r. medialis nervi supraorbitalis
 r. medialis rami posterioris nervi cervicalis
 r. medialis rami posterioris nervi lumbalis
 r. medialis rami posterioris nervi sacralis
 r. medialis rami posterioris nervi thoracici
 r. membranae tympani nervi auriculotemporalis
 r. meningeus nervi mandibularis
 r. meningeus nervi maxillaris
 r. meningeus nervi spinalis
 r. meningeus nervi vagi
 r. meningeus recurrens nervi ophthalmici
 rami mentales nervi mentalis
 r. muscularis
 rami musculares nervi axillaris
 rami musculares nervi femoralis
 rami musculares nervi fibularis profundi
 rami musculares nervi fibularis superficialis
 rami musculares nervorum intercostalium
 rami musculares nervi ischiadici
 rami musculares nervi mediani

ramus *(continued)*
 rami musculares nervi musculocutanei
 rami musculares nervi peronei profundi
 rami musculares nervi peronei superficialis
 rami musculares nervi radialis
 rami musculares nervi tibialis
 rami musculares nervi ulnaris
 rami musculares plexus lumbalis
 rami musculares rami anterioris nervi obturatorii
 rami musculares rami externi nervi accessorii
 rami musculares rami posterioris nervi obturatorii
 r. musculi stylopharyngei nervi glossopharyngei
 r. nasalis externus nervi ethmoidalis anterioris
 rami nasales externi nervi infraorbitalis
 rami nasales interni laterales nervi ethmoidalis anterioris
 rami nasales interni mediales nervi ethmoidalis anterioris
 rami nasales interni nervi ethmoidalis anterioris
 rami nasales interni nervi infraorbitalis
 rami nasales nervi ethmoidalis anterioris
 rami nasales posteriores inferiores nervi palatini majoris
 rami nasales posteriores superiores laterales nervi maxillaris
 rami nasales posteriores superiores mediales nervi maxillaris

ramus *(continued)*

r. nervi oculomotorii ad ganglii ciliare

r. occipitalis nervi auricularis posterioris

rami oesophageales gangliorum thoracicorum

rami oesophagei nervi laryngei recurrentis

rami orbitales ganglii pterygopalatini

rami orbitales nervi maxillaris

r. palmaris nervi mediani

r. palmaris nervi ulnaris

rami palpebrales inferiores nervi infraorbitalis

rami palpebrales nervi infratrochlearis

rami parotidei nervi auriculotemporalis

r. pericardiacus nervi phrenici

rami perineales nervi cutanei femoris posterioris

r. pharyngeus ganglii pterygopalatini

rami pharyngei nervi glossopharyngei

rami pharyngei nervi laryngei recurrentis

r. pharyngeus nervi vagi

rami phrenicoabdominales nervi phrenici

r. posterior nervi auricularis magni

rami posteriores nervorum cervicalium

r. posterior nervi coccygei

r. posterior nervi cutanei antebrachii medialis

rami posteriores nervorum lumbalium

r. posterior nervi obturatorii

rami posteriores nervorum sacralium

r. posterior nervi spinalis

ramus *(continued)*

rami posteriores nervorum thoracicorum

r. posterior sulci lateralis cerebri

r. profundus nervi plantaris lateralis

r. profundus nervi radialis

r. profundus nervi ulnaris

rami pulmonales plexus pulmonalis

rami pulmonales thoracici gangliorum thoracicorum

r. recurrens nervi spinalis

r. renalis nervi splanchnici minoris

rami renales nervi vagi

rami renales plexus coeliaci

r. sinus carotici nervi glossopharyngei

r. stylohyoideus nervi facialis

r. superficialis nervi plantaris lateralis

r. superficialis nervi radialis

r. superficialis nervi ulnaris

r. superior nervi oculomotorii

rami superiores nervi transversi colli

r. sympatheticus ganglii ciliaris

r. sympathicus ganglii ciliaris

r. sympathicus ad ganglion submandibulare

rami temporales nervi facialis

rami temporales superficiales nervi auriculotemporalis

r. tentorii nervi ophthalmici

r. thyrohyoideus ansae cervicalis

rami tonsillares nervi glossopharyngei

ramus *(continued)*
>   rami tonsillares nervorum palatinorum minorum
>   rami tracheales nervi laryngei recurrentis
>   rami tracheales nervi recurrentis
>   r. tubalis plexus tympanici
>   r. tubarius plexus tympanici
>   rami ventrales nervorum cervicalium
>   r. ventralis nervi coccygei
>   rami ventrales nervorum lumbalium
>   ventral rami of thoracic nerves
>   rami ventrales nervorum sacralium
>   r. ventralis nervi spinalis
>   rami ventrales nervorum thoracicorum
>   r. visceralis
>   rami zygomatici nervi facialis
>   r. zygomaticofacialis nervi zygomatici
>   r. zygomaticotemporalis nervi zygomatici

Ranvier
>   internode of R.
>   nodes of R.
>   R's tactile disks

ranine

raphe
>   r. corporis callosi
>   r. of corpus callosum
>   median r. of medulla oblongata
>   r. mediana medullae oblongatae
>   median r. of pons
>   r. mediana pontina
>   r. medullae oblongatae
>   r. pontis

RAS
>   reticular activating system

rasagiline

Rasmussen
>   bundle of R.
>   R's nerve fibers
>   olivocochlear bundle of R.

Rathke
>   R's cleft cysts
>   R's cysts
>   R's pouch tumor
>   R's tumor

Raymond
>   R's apoplexy
>   R.-Cestan syndrome

react

reaction
>   axon r.
>   axonal r.
>   Bekhterev's (Bechterew's) r.
>   cadaveric r.
>   consensual r.
>   Marchi's r.
>   pain r.
>   startle r.
>   tendon r.

reactivity

Rebif

rebound
>   analgesic r. headache
>   REM r.

reception

receptor
>   adrenergic r's
> α-adrenergic r's
> β-adrenergic r's
>   alpha r's
> γ-aminobutyric acid r's
>   beta r's
>   cholinergic r's
>   cold r.
>   contact r.
>   cutaneous r.
>   distance r.

receptor *(continued)*
    GABA r's
    gustatory r.
    hair follicle r's
    Iggo r.
    J-r's
    joint r.
    juxtapulmonary r's
    muscarinic r's
    muscle r.
    N_1-r's
    N_2-r's
    nicotinic r's
    nonadapting r.
    olfactory r.
    opiate r.
    opioid r.
    pain r.
    pressure r.
    rapidly adapting r.
    sensory r.
    slowly adapting r.
    stretch r.
    tactile r.
    thermal r.
    touch r.
    vibration r.
    warmth r.
recess
    chiasmatic r.
    r. of interpeduncular fossa,
      anterior
    r. of interpeduncular fossa,
      posterior
    Tarin's r.
    triangular r.
    infundibular r.
    lateral r. of fourth ventricle
    supraoptic r.
    optic r.
    pineal r.
    suprapineal r.
recessus
    r. infundibularis
    r. infundibuli
    r. lateralis ventriculi quarti
    r. opticus
    r. pinealis

recessus *(continued)*
    r. supraopticus
    r. suprapinealis
recruitment
redecussate
Recklinghausen's disease
Redlich-Fisher miliary plaques
reflex
    abdominal r's
    abdominocardiac r.
    Abrams' heart r.
    Achilles tendon r.
    adductor r. of foot
    adductor r. of thigh
    allied r's
    anal r.
    ankle r.
    antagonistic r's
    anticus r.
    antigravity r's
    attitudinal r's
    audito-oculogyric r.
    auditory r.
    auriculocervical nerve r.
    auriculopalpebral r.
    axon r.
    Babinski's r.
    bar r.
    Barkman's r.
    basal joint r.
    Bechterew's r.
    Bekhterev's r.
    Bekhterev's deep r.
    Bekhterev-Mendel r.
    biceps r.
    bladder r.
    blepharocardiac r.
    blink r.
    brachioradialis r.
    Brain's r.
    brain stem r's
    Brissaud's r.
    Brudzinski's r.
    bulbocavernosus r.
    bulbomimic r.
    bulbospongiosus r.
    Chaddock's r.

reflex *(continued)*
- chain r.
- chin r.
- ciliospinal r.
- clasp-knife r.
- closed loop r.
- cochleopupillary r.
- concealed r.
- consensual r.
- convulsive r.
- coordinated r.
- corneomandibular r.
- corneomental r.
- corneopterygoid r.
- cranial r.
- cremasteric r.
- crossed r.
- crossed adductor r.
- crossed extension r.
- cuboidodigital r.
- cutaneous pupillary r.
- dartos r.
- deep r.
- delayed r.
- depressor r.
- digital r.
- doll's eye r.
- dorsal r.
- dorsocuboidal r.
- elbow r.
- epigastric r.
- Erben's r.
- erector spinae r.
- Escherich's r.
- external auditory meatus r.
- facial r.
- faucial r.
- femoral r.
- finger-to-nose r.
- finger-thumb r.
- flexion r.
- flexor r., paradoxical
- front-tap r.
- gag r.
- Geigel's r.
- glabellar r.
- gluteal r.
- Gordon's r.

reflex *(continued)*
- grasp r.
- grasping r.
- gustolacrimal r.
- H-r.
- heart r.
- heel-knee-shin r.
- heel-tap r.
- Hirschberg's r.
- Hoffmann's r.
- Hughes' r.
- hypochondrial r.
- hypogastric r.
- indirect r.
- infraspinatus r.
- inguinal r.
- interscapular r.
- inverted radial r.
- jaw r.
- jaw jerk r.
- Joffroy's r.
- Juster r.
- Kehrer's r.
- Kisch's r.
- knee jerk r.
- Kocher's r.
- labyrinthine r's
- laughter r.
- local r.
- Lovén r.
- lumbar r.
- Lust's r.
- McCarthy's r.
- McCormac's r.
- Magnus and de Kleijn neck r's
- mandibular r.
- Marinesco-Radovici r.
- mass r.
- Mayer's r.
- Mendel's r.
- Mendel-Bekhterev r.
- micturition r.
- Mondonesi's r.
- Morley's peritoneocutaneous r.
- nasal r.
- nasomental r.
- Mendel's dorsal r. of foot

reflex *(continued)*
    neck r's
    nociceptive r's
    obliquus r.
    oculoauricular r.
    oculocephalogyric r.
    oculorespiratory r.
    open loop r.
    Oppenheim's r.
    orienting r.
    palmar r.
    palm-chin r.
    palmomental r.
    paradoxical pupillary r.
    patellar r.
    patelloadductor r.
    pectoral r.
    penile r.
    penis r.
    perianal r.
    periosteal r.
    pharyngeal r.
    phasic r.
    Philippson's r.
    plantar r.
    platysmal r.
    pollicomental r.
    postural r.
    pouting r.
    proprioceptive r.
    psychogalvanic r.
    Puusepp's r.
    quadriceps r.
    quadrupedal extensor r.
    radial r.
    regional r.
    Remak's r.
    Riddoch's mass r.
    righting r.
    Rossolimo's r.
    Ruggeri's r.
    Saenger's r.
    scapular r.
    scapulohumeral r.
    Schäffer's r.
    scratch r.
    scrotal r.
    segmental r.
    sexual r.

reflex *(continued)*
    simple r.
    skin r.
    skin pupillary r.
    Snellen's r.
    sole r.
    somatointestinal r.
    spinal r.
    startle r.
    static r.
    statotonic r's
    Stookey's r.
    Strümpell's r.
    sucking r.
    superficial r.
    supinator longus r.
    supraorbital r.
    suprapatellar r.
    suprapubic r.
    supraumbilical r.
    tarsophalangeal r.
    tendon r.
    testicular compression r.
    threat r.
    Throckmorton's r.
    tibioadductor r.
    toe r.
    tonic r.
    triceps r.
    triceps surae r.
    ulnar r.
    urinary r.
    vagus r.
    vesical r.
    vestibular r's
    virile r.
    visceral r.
    withdrawal r.
    zygomatic r.

reflexogenic

reflexogenous

reflexograph

reflexology

reflexometer

reflexophil

Refsum disease

regio *pl.* regiones
  r. hypothalamica anterior
  r. hypothalamica dorsalis
  r. hypothalamica intermedia
  r. hypothalamica lateralis
  r. hypothalamica posterior

region
  Broca's r.
  extrapolar r.
  hypothalamic r., anterior
  hypothalamic r., intermediate
  hypothalamic r., lateral
  hypothalamic r., posterior
  infundibulotubular r.
  mammillary r.
  motor r.
  opticostriate r.
  prefrontal r.
  preoptic r.
  pretectal r.
  rolandic r.
  sensory r's
  supraoptic r.
  hypothalamic r., dorsal

Reichert
  R's substance
  substantia innominata of R.

Reil
  insula of R.
  island of R.
  ribbon of R.
  substantia innominata of R.
  R's sulcus
  taeniola corporis callosi of R.
  R's triangle
  trigone of R.

Reilly bodies

reinnervation

REM
  rapid eye movements
    REM latency
    REM rebound
    REM sleep

REM *(continued)*
    REM sleep behavior disorder

Remak
  R's ganglion
  R's paralysis
  R's reflex
  R's sign
  R's symptom

Renaut's bodies

Renshaw cells

repolarization

Requip

reservoir
  Ommaya r.

response
  auditory visual-evoked r's
  blink r's
  cold r., paradoxical
  decremental r.
  decrementing r.
  F r.
  galvanic skin r.
  H r.
  incremental r.
  M r.
  orienting r.
  relaxation r.

retardation
  psychomotor r.

rete *pl.* retia
  r. mirabile

reticular activating system (RAS)

reticulopituicyte

retinotopic

retrobulbar

retrochiasmatic

retrocochlear

retrocollis

retrocursive

retrogasserian

retropulsion

Rett syndrome

Retzius' foramen

reuptake

reverberation

Revilliod's sign

Rexed's laminae

Reye
R. syndrome
R.-like syndrome

rheobase

rheonome

rhesus

rhigosis

rhigotic

rhinencephalon

rhinocele

rhinocoele

rhinorrhea
cerebrospinal fluid r.

rhizolysis

rhizomeningomyelitis

rhizotomy
anterior r.
chemical r.
dorsal r.
glycerol r.
percutaneous r.
percutaneous radiofre-
quency r.
posterior r.
retrogasserian r.
trigeminal r.

rhombencephalon

rhombocoele

rhythm
alpha r.
Berger r.
beta r.
delta r.
gamma r.
mu r.
theta r.

ribbon
r. of Reil

right-handed

rigidity
catatonic r.
clasp-knife r.
cogwheel r.
decerebrate r.
hemiplegic r.
lead-pipe r.
paratonic r.

Riley-Day syndrome

Rilutek

rimula

RIND
reversible ischemic neurologic defect

ring
atrial r.

Rinne test

Ritalin
R. SR

Ritscher-Schinzel syndrome

Robert's syndrome

rod
olfactory r.

Rohon-Beard cells

rolandic angle

Rolando
angle of R.
R's cells
fissure of R.

Rolando *(continued)*
    R's gelatinous substance
    tubercle of R.
    R's zone

Roller's nucleus

Romberg
    R's sign
    R's spasm
    R's test

rombergism

roof
    r. of fourth ventricle
    r. of lateral ventricle
    r. of third ventricle

root
    r's of ansa cervicalis
    anterior r. of ansa cervicalis
    anterior r. of spinal nerve
    r's of brachial plexus
    cochlear r. of vestibulocochlear nerve
    cranial r. of accessory nerve
    dorsal r. of spinal nerve
    facial r.
    r. of facial nerve
    inferior r. of ansa cervicalis
    inferior r. of vestibulocochlear nerve
    lateral r. of median nerve
    lateral r. of optic tract
    long r. of ciliary ganglion
    medial r. of median nerve
    medial r. of optic tract
    motor r. of ciliary ganglion
    motor r. of mandibular nerve
    motor r. of spinal nerve
    motor r. of submandibular ganglion
    motor r. of trigeminal nerve
    nasociliary r. of ciliary ganglion
    nerve r's
    nerve r., motor

root *(continued)*
    nerve r., sensory
    oculomotor r. of ciliary ganglion
    r. of otic ganglion
    parasympathetic r. of ciliary ganglion
    parasympathetic r. of otic ganglion
    parasympathetic r. of pterygopalatine ganglion
    parasympathetic r. of sublingual ganglion
    parasympathetic r. of submandibular ganglion
    posterior r. of ansa cervicalis
    posterior r. of spinal nerve
    sensory r. of ciliary ganglion
    sensory r. of mandibular nerve
    sensory r. of otic ganglion
    sensory r. of pterygopalatine ganglion
    sensory r. of spinal nerve
    sensory r. of submandibular ganglion
    sensory r. of trigeminal nerve
    short r. of ciliary ganglion
    spinal r's
    spinal r. of accessory nerve
    r's of spinal nerves
    superior r. of ansa cervicalis
    superior r. of vestibulocochlear nerve
    sympathetic r. of ciliary ganglion
    sympathetic r. of pterygopalatine ganglion
    ventral r. of spinal nerve
    vestibular r. of vestibulocochlear nerve

rootlet
    r's of spinal nerve

ropinirole

Rosenbach's sign

Rosenberg-Chutorian syndrome

Rosenthal
R's degeneration
R. fibers

Rossolimo
R's reflex
R's sign

rostrum *pl.* rostra
r. corporis callosi

Roth (Rot)
R's disease
R's syndrome
R.-Bernhardt disease
R.-Bernhardt syndrome

Roussy
R.-Dejerine syndrome
R.-Lévy syndrome

Rubenstein-Taybi syndrome

rubric

rubrospinal

rubrothalamic

Ruffini
R's brush
R's corpuscle
R's cylinder
R's ending
R's organ

Ruggeri
R's reflex
R's sign

Rukavina
R's syndrome
R. type familial amyloid
polyneuropathy

rule
Allen's r.
Bergmann's r.
dermatomal r.
Jackson's r.

Russian
R. autumnal encephalitis
R. endemic encephalitis
R. forest-spring encephalitis
R. spring-summer encephalitis
R. tick-borne encephalitis
R. vernal encephalitis

S
  S sleep

Sabril

Saethre-Chotzen syndrome

St. Anthony's dance

St. Guy's dance

St. John's dance

St. Louis encephalitis

St. Vitus' dance

Sala's cells

Sandifer syndrome

saltation

saltatorial

saltatoric

saltatory

sand
  brain s.

Sanfilippo syndrome

Sanger Brown ataxia

sapophore

SI area

SII area

sarcoma
  reticulum cell s. of the
    brain

satellitosis

Saturday night palsy

scale
  Glasgow Coma S.
  Glasgow Outcome S.

Scarpa
  S's ganglion
  S's nerve

scatophagy

scelotyrbe

Schäffer's reflex

Scheie syndrome

Scherer's secondary structures

Schilder
  S's disease
  S's encephalitis

Schinzel-Giedion syndrome

Schirmer's syndrome

schistorachis

schizaxon

schizencephalic

schizencephaly

schizogyria

schizophasia

schizophrenia
  acute s.
  ambulatory s.
  borderline s.
  catatonic s.
  disorganized s.
  hebephrenic s.
  latent s.
  paranoid s.
  prepsychotic s.
  process s.
  pseudoneurotic s.
  pseudopsychopathic s.
  reactive s.
  residual s.
  schizoaffective s.
  simple s.
  undifferentiated s.

schizophrenic

schizophreniform

schnauzkrampf

Schlesinger
  S's phenomenon
  S's sign

Schlösser's treatment

Schmidt
    S's syndrome
    S.-Lanterman clefts
    S.-Lanterman incisures

Schmiedel's ganglion

Scholz's disease

Schramm's phenomenon

Schreiber's maneuver

Schroeder van der Kolk's law

Schultze
    S's cells
    comma tract of S.
    S's sign
    S's tract
    S.-Chvostek sign

Schütz
    S's bundle
    S's fasciculus
    S's tract

Schwalbe
    S's fissure
    S's foramen
    S's nucleus

Schwann
    S. cell
    S. cell tumor
    S's membrane
    S's nucleus

schwannoglioma

schwannoma
    acoustic s.

schwannomin

schwannosis

Schwartz-Jampel syndrome

sciatica

sclerencephalia

sclerencephaly

sclérose en plaques

sclerosis
    amyotrophic lateral s.
    anterolateral s.
    combined s.
    concentric s.
    diffuse s.
    diffuse cerebral s.
    disseminated s.
    Erb's s.
    familial centrolobar s.
    focal s.
    hippocampal s.
    insular s.
    lateral s.
    lobar s.
    mesial temporal s.
    multiple s.
    Pelizaeus-Merzbacher s.
    posterior s.
    posterior spinal s.
    posterolateral s.
    primary lateral s.
    ventrolateral s.

scombroid

score
    Kurtzke s.
    stroke s.

scotodinia

scotoma
    flittering s.
    scintillating s.

secretomotor

secretomotory

segment
    initial s.
    interannular s.
    internodal s.
    medullary s.
    neural s.
    Ranvier's s.
    Schmidt-Lanterman s.
    spinal s's
    s's of spinal cord

segmentum
    segmenta cervicalia [1–8]

segmentum *(continued)*
    segmenta coccygea [1–3]
    segmenta lumbalia [1–5]
    segmenta lumbaria
    segmenta medullae spinalis
    segmenta sacralia [1–5]
    segmenta thoracica [1–12]

Séguin
    S's sign
    S's signal symptom

Seitelberger's disease

seizure
    absence s.
    adversive s.
    astatic s.
    atonic s.
    atypical absence s.
    auditory s.
    automatic s.
    centrencephalic s.
    clonic s.
    complex partial s.
    drop s.
    drug-withdrawal s.
    electrographic s.
    febrile s's
    focal s.
    focal motor s.
    generalized anoxic s.
    generalized febrile s.
    generalized tonic-clonic s.
    grand mal s.
    hypoglycemic s.
    jackknife s's
    jacksonian s.
    multifocal s.
    myoclonic s.
    myoclonic-astatic s.
    neonatal s.
    partial s.
    petit mal s.
    postischemic s.
    postpump s.
    psychogenic s.
    psychomotor s.
    pyridoxine-deficiency s.
    reflex s.

seizure *(continued)*
    rolandic s.
    salaam s's
    sensory s.
    serial s's
    simple partial s.
    somatosensory s.
    sound-sensitive s.
    subtle s.
    tonic s.
    tonic-clonic s.
    uncinate s.
    unclassified epileptic s.
    unilateral s.
    vestibulogenic s.
    visual s.

selachian

sella
    empty s.
    s. turcica

Semliki Forest encephalitis

sellar

semicoma

semicomatose

semidecussation

semiplegia

sensation
    cincture s.
    cutaneous s.
    delayed s.
    general s.
    girdle s.
    objective s.
    pin s.
    primary s.
    referred s.
    reflex s.
    secondary s.
    subjective s.
    transferred s.
    vascular s.

sense
    body s.
    chemical s.

sense *(continued)*
    contact s.
    distance s.
    s. of equilibrium
    external s.
    internal s.
    joint s.
    kinesthetic s.
    labyrinthine s.
    motion s.
    movement s.
    muscle s.
    muscular s.
    pain s.
    position s.
    posture s.
    pressure s.
    proprioceptive s.
    seventh s.
    sixth s.
    somatic s's
    space s.
    special s's
    static s.
    tactile s.
    temperature s.
    vestibular s.
    vibration s.
    visceral s.

sensibility
    bone s.
    common s.
    deep s.
    epicritic s.
    joint s.
    mesoblastic s.
    pallesthetic s.
    palmesthetic s.
    proprioceptive s.
    protopathic s.
    splanchnesthetic s.
    vibratory s.

sensibilization

sensible

sensiferous

sensigenous

sensimeter

sensitive

sensitivity
    proportional s.

sensomotor

sensorial

sensoriglandular

sensorimotor

sensorimuscular

sensorineural

sensorium
    s. commune

sensorivascular

sensorivasomotor

sensory

sentient

septineuritis
    Nicolau's s.

septum *pl.* septa
    cervical s., intermediate
    s. cervicale intermedium
    s. lucidum
    median s. of spinal cord, dorsal
    median s. of spinal cord, posterior
    s. medianum dorsale medullae spinalis
    s. medianum posterius medullae spinalis
    s. pellucidum
    precommissural s.
    s. precommissurale
    subarachnoidal s.
    s. verum

serotonergic

serotonin

serotoninergic

servomechanism

shark
  Greenland s.
  soupfin s.

sheath
  arachnoid s.
  dural s.
  external s. of optic nerve
  fibrous s. of optic nerve
  s. of Henle
  inner s. of optic nerve
  internal s. of optic nerve
  s. of Key and Retzius
  lamellar s.
  Mauthner's s.
  medullary s.
  myelin s.
  nerve s.
  neurilemmal s.
  s's of optic nerve
  outer s. of optic nerve
  perivascular s.
  pial s.
  s. of Schwann

Sherrington
  S's law
  S's phenomenon

shiver

shivering

shock
  spinal s.

Shprintzen-Goldberg syndrome

shunt
  lumboperitoneal s.
  Torkildsen's s.
  ventriculoatrial s.
  ventriculocisternal s.
  ventriculoperitoneal s.
  ventriculopleural s.
  ventriculovenous s.

sickness
  laughing s.

Shy-Drager syndrome

Sicard's syndrome

Siemerling's nucleus

sign
  Abadie's s.
  André Thomas s.
  anterior tibial s.
  anticus s.
  Babinski's s.
  Babinski's toe s.
  Baillarger's s.
  Bamberger's s.
  Barré's s.
  Barré's pyramidal s.
  Bastian-Bruns' s.
  Battle's s.
  Beevor's s.
  Bekhterev's s.
  Bell's s.
  Berger's s.
  Biernacki's s.
  Bonnet's s.
  Bordier-Fränkel s.
  Bragard's s.
  Brown-Séquard's s.
  Brudzinski's s.
  Bruns' s.
  Cantelli's s.
  Chaddock's s.
  Charcot's s.
  Chvostek's s.
  Claude's hyperkinesis s.
  Chvostek-Weiss s.
  cogwheel s.
  complementary opposi-
    tion s.
  contralateral s.
  coughing s.
  Crichton-Browne's s.
  Crowe's s.
  Dejerine's s.
  Demianoff's s.
  doll's eye s.
  DTP s.
  Duckworth's s.
  echo s.
  Erben's s.
  Escherich's s.
  external malleolar s.
  facial s.

sign *(continued)*
    Fajersztajn's crossed sciat-
        ic s.
    fan s.
    forearm s.
    formication s.
    Fränkel's s.
    Froment's paper s.
    Goldthwait's s.
    Gordon's s.
    Gowers' s.
    Grasset's s.
    Grasset-Bychowski s.
    Grasset-Gaussel-Hoover s.
    Guilland's s.
    Gunn's s.
    Hahn's s.
    Heilbronner's s.
    Hirschberg's s.
    Hitzelberger's s.
    Hochsinger's s.
    Hoffmann's s.
    Holmes' s.
    Hoover's s.
    Horsley's s.
    Huntington's s.
    hyperkinesis s.
    interossei s.
    jugular s.
    Kernig's s.
    Kerr's s.
    Kleist's s.
    Klippel-Weil s.
    Lafora's s.
    Lasègue's s.
    leg s.
    Leichtenstern's s.
    Léri's s.
    Lhermitte's s.
    Linder's s.
    Livierato's s.
    Lust's s.
    Macewen's s.
    Marie-Foix s.
    Marinesco's s.
    Mendel-Bekhterev s.
    Minor's s.
    Myerson's s.
    neck s.

sign *(continued)*
    Negro's s.
    Neri's s.
    Oppenheim's s.
    orbicularis s.
    Parkinson's s.
    Parrot's s.
    Pende's s.
    peroneal s.
    Piotrowski's s.
    Pitres' s.
    Pool-Schlesinger s.
    Prévost's s.
    pronation s.
    pyramid s.
    pyramidal s.
    Queckenstedt's s.
    radialis s.
    Radovici's s.
    Remak's s.
    reservoir s.
    Revilliod's s.
    Romberg's s.
    Rosenbach's s.
    Rossolimo's s.
    Ruggeri's s.
    Saenger's s.
    Schlesinger's s.
    Schultze's s.
    Schultze-Chvostek s.
    Séguin's s.
    setting-sun s.
    Simon's s.
    Souques' s.
    stairs s.
    Stewart-Holmes s.
    Strümpell's s.
    Theimich's lip s.
    Thomas' s.
    Throckmorton's s.
    tibialis s.
    Tinel's s.
    toe s.
    Trousseau's s.
    Turyn's s.
    Vanzetti's s.
    Wartenberg's s.
    Westphal's s.

silence
    electrical s.
    electrocerebral s.

siliqua
    s. olivae

Simmerlin's dystrophy

Simon's sign

simultagnosia

simultanagnosia

Sinemet

sinistral

sinistrality

sinistrocerebral

sinistromanual

sinistropedal

sinus
    Breschet's s.
    s. cavernosus
    cavernous s.
    circular s.
    s. circularis
    cranial s's
    dermal s.
    s's of dura mater
    s. durae matris
    dural s's
    s. intercavernosus anterior
    s. intercavernosus poste-
        rior
    lateral s.
    longitudinal s., inferior
    longitudinal s., superior
    marginal s's
    s. marginalis
    occipital s.
    s. occipitalis
    parasinoidal s's
    petrosal s., inferior
    petrosal s., superior
    s. petrosus inferior
    s. petrosus superior
    s. rectus

sinus (continued)
    rhomboid s. of Henle
    Ridley's s.
    sagittal s., inferior
    sagittal s., superior
    s. sagittalis inferior
    s. sagittalis superior
    sigmoid s.
    s. sigmoideus
    sphenoparietal s.
    s. sphenoparietalis
    straight s.
    subarachnoidal s's
    tentorial s.
    transverse s. of dura mater
    s. transversus durae matris
    s. venosi durales
    venous s's of dura mater
    intercavernous s., anterior
    intercavernous s., posterior
    s. petrosquamosus
    petrosquamous s.

Sjögren
    S. syndrome
    S.-Larsson syndrome

skeletal

skeleton

skull
    cloverleaf s.

sleep
    active s.
    D s.
    deep s.
    desynchronized s.
    dreaming s.
    fast wave s.
    non-rapid eye movement s.
    NREM s.
    orthodox s.
    paradoxical s.
    paroxysmal s.
    quiet s.
    rapid eye movement s.
    REM s.
    S s.
    slow wave s.
    synchronized s.

Sluder
    S's neuralgia
    S's syndrome

smell

smell-brain

Smith-Lemli-Opitz syndrome

SNAP
    sensory nerve action potential

Sneddon's syndrome

Snellen's reflex

softening
    s. of the brain
    hemorrhagic s.
    pyriform s.
    red s.
    white s.
    yellow s.

solar
    s. plexus

somatesthesia

somatesthetic

somatochrome

somatognosis

somatomotor

somatosensory

somatotopagnosia

somatotopic

somesthesia

somesthetic

somnocinematograph

somnolence

somnolent

somnolentia

sopor

soporous

sound
    cracked-pot s.
    cranial, cracked-pot s.

Souques
    S's phenomenon
    S's sign

space
    epicerebral s.
    epidural s.
    epispinal s.
    extradural s.
    His' perivascular s's
    intercrural s.
    interpeduncular s.
    intervaginal s's of optic
      nerve
    Magendie's s's
    Marie's quadrilateral s.
    Meckel's s.
    parasinoidal s's
    perforated s., anterior
    perforated s., posterior
    perineuronal s.
    perivascular s's
    quadrilateral s. of Marie
    Schwalbe's s's
    subarachnoid s.
    subdural s.
    subepicranial s.
    Tarin's s.
    Virchow-Robin s's

spasm
    athetoid s.
    Bell's s.
    carpopedal s.
    clonic s.
    dancing s.
    facial s.
    fixed s.
    glottic s.
    habit s.
    hemifacial s.
    histrionic s.
    infantile s's

spasm *(continued)*
  infantile massive s's
  intention s.
  jackknife s's
  lock s.
  malleatory s.
  massive s.
  mixed s.
  mobile s.
  myopathic s.
  phonatory s.
  progressive torsion s.
  Romberg's s.
  salaam s's
  saltatory s.
  tetanic s.
  tonic s.
  tonoclonic s.
  torsion s.
  toxic s.

spasmodic

spasmogen

spasmogenic

spasmolysis

spasmophile

spasmophilic

spasmus

spastic

spasticity
  clasp-knife s.

spatium *pl.* spatia
  s. epidurale
  s. extradurale
  spatia intervaginalia nervi
    optici
  s. leptomeningeum
  s. peridurale
  s. subarachnoideum
  s. subdurale

specificity
  neuronal s.

SPECT
  single photon emission
    computed tomography

spectroscopy
  magnetic resonance s.
    (MRS)

spectrum *pl.* spectra
  fortification s.

speech
  echo s.
  staccato s.
  telegraphic s.

spherule
  s's of Fulci

sphingolipidosis

spike
  end-plate s's
  s.-and-wave pattern

spina *pl.* spinae
  s. bifida
  s. bifida anterior
  s. bifida aperta
  s. bifida cystica
  s. bifida manifesta
  s. bifida occulta
  s. bifida posterior

spinal

spindle
  muscle s.
  neuromuscular s.
  neurotendinous s.
  sleep s's
  tendon s.

spine
  cleft s.
  dendritic s.

spinifugal

spinipetal

spinobulbar

spinocerebellar

spinocerebellum

spinocortical

spinogalvanization

spinopetal

spinotectal

spinothalamic

spinovestibular
s. tract

spiral
Perroncito's s's

Spitzka
column of S. and Lissauer
S's nucleus
S's tract
S.-Lissauer tract

splanchnesthesia

splanchnesthetic

splanchnicectomy

splanchnicotomy

splenial

splenium
s. corporis callosi

spondyloschisis

spondylosis
cervical s.
s. deformans

spongioblastoma
s. multiforme
polar s.
s. polare
unipolar s.
s. unipolare

spongiocyte

spongiocytoma

spot
cold s.
hot s.
hypnogenetic s.

spot (continued)
pain s's
temperature s's
Trousseau's s.
warm s's

spur
Morand's s.
calcarine s.

Staderini's nucleus

stage
s's of sleep

stalk
cerebellar s.
hypophysial s.
infundibular s.
neural s.
pineal s.
pituitary s.
s's of thalamus

state
alpha s.
anelectrotonic s.
catelectrotonic s.
central excitatory s.
de-efferented s.
dreamy s.
hypnagogic s.
hypnopompic s.
local excitatory s.
persistent vegetative s.
refractory s.
twilight s.

status
absence s.
s. choreicus
complex partial s.
s. convulsivus
s. cribalis
s. cribrosus
s. criticus
s. dysmyelinatus
s. dysmyelinisatus
s. epilepticus
s. hemicranicus
s. lacunaris
s. lacunosus
s. marmoratus

status *(continued)*
    s. migrainosus
    s. epilepticus, nonconvul-
        sive
    petit mal s.
    psychomotor s.
    simple partial s.
    s. epilepticus, tonic-clonic
    s. verrucosus
    s. vertiginosus
    s. epilepticus, convulsive

stauroplegia

steal
    subclavian s.

Steele-Richardson-Olszewski
    syndrome

Stein-Leventhal syndrome

stellectomy

stem
    brain s.
    infundibular s.

stenosis
    spinal s.

stereoagnosis

stereoanesthesia

stereocognosy

stereoencephalotome

stereoencephalotomy

stereognosis

stereognostic

stereotactic

stereotaxic

stereotaxis

stereotaxy

stethoparalysis

stethospasm

Stevens-Johnson syndrome

Stewart-Holmes sign

Stickler syndrome

Stilling
    S's column
    S's fibers
    S's nucleus

stimulate

stimulation
    areal s.
    audio-visual-tactile s.
    functional neuromuscu-
        lar s.
    nonspecific s.
    paradoxical s.
    paraspecific s.
    photic s.
    punctual s.
    repetitive nerve s.
    transcutaneous electrical
        nerve s. (TENS)
    transcutaneous nerve s.
        (TNS)

stimulator
    electronic s.
    vagus nerve s. (VNS)

stimulus *pl.* stimuli
    adequate s.
    chemical s.
    electric s.
    heterologous s.
    homologous s.
    liminal s.
    maximal s.
    mechanical s.
    patterned s.
    subliminal s.
    subthreshold s.
    supraliminal s.
    supramaximal s.
    suprathreshold s.
    threshold s.

Stookey's reflex

strangalesthesia

stratum *pl.* strata
    s. cinereum

stratum *(continued)*
    strata colliculi rostralis
    s. ganglionare nervi optici
    ganglionic s. of optic nerve
    s. granulosum cerebelli
    strata grisea et alba collic-
        uli rostralis
    strata grisea et alba collic-
        uli superioris
    s. griseum intermedium
        colliculi superioris
    s. griseum profundum col-
        liculi superioris
    s. griseum superficiale col-
        liculi superioris
    s. lacunosum
    s. lemnisci
    strata colliculi superioris
    s. lucidum hippocampi
    s. medullare intermedium
        colliculi superioris
    s. medullare profundum
        colliculi superioris
    s. moleculare cerebelli
    s. moleculare hippocampi
    s. neuronorum piriformium
    s. opticum colliculi superi-
        oris
    s. oriens hippocampi
    s. plexiforme cerebelli
    s. purkinjense cerebelli
    s. pyramidale hippocampi
    s. radiatum hippocampi
    s. zonale colliculi superi-
        oris
    s. zonale thalami

streak
    meningitic s.

strephosymbolia

stria *pl.* striae
    acoustic striae
    auditory striae
    Baillarger's external s.
    Baillarger's inner s.
    Baillarger's internal s.
    Baillarger's outer s.
    s. diagonalis

stria *(continued)*
    s. diagonalis (Broca)
    external s. of Baillarger
    s. of external granular layer
    s. of Gennari
    inner s. of Baillarger
    internal s. of Baillarger
    s. of internal granular layer
    s. of internal pyramidal
        layer
    Kaes' s.
    Kaes-Bekhterev s.
    s. laminae granularis exter-
        nae
    s. laminae granularis inter-
        nae
    s. laminae molecularis
    s. laminae plexiformis
    s. laminae pyramidalis in-
        ternae
    s. of Lanci
    longitudinal s. of corpus
        callosum, lateral
    longitudinal s. of corpus
        callosum, medial
    s. longitudinalis lateralis
        corporis callosi
    s. longitudinalis medialis
        corporis callosi
    striae medullares acusticae
    striae medullares fossae
        rhomboideae
    s. medullaris thalami
    striae medullares ventriculi
        quarti
    medullary s. of corpus
        striatum, lateral
    medullary s. of corpus
        striatum, medial
    medullary striae of fourth
        ventricle
    medullary striae of rhom-
        boid fossa
    medullary s. of thalamus
    meningitic s.
    s. of molecular layer
    striae olfactoriae
    s. olfactoria lateralis
    s. olfactoria medialis

stria *(continued)*
    olfactory striae
    olfactory s., intermediate
    olfactory striae, lateral
    olfactory s., medial
    outer s. of Baillarger
    s. terminalis
    transverse striae of corpus
      callosum

striae *(plural of* stria)

striatal

striatonigral

striatum

striocerebellar

striomotor

strionigral

stripe
    Baillarger's external s.
    Baillarger's inner s.
    Baillarger's internal s.
    Baillarger's outer s.
    external s. of Baillarger
    s. of Gennari
    inner s. of Baillarger
    internal s. of Baillarger
    outer s. of Baillarger
    Vicq d'Azyr's s.

stroke
    completed s.
    developing s.
    embolic s.
    s. in evolution
    ischemic s.
    paralytic s.
    progressing s.
    thrombotic s.

stroma *pl.* stromata
    s. ganglii
    s. ganglionicum

structure
    Scherer's secondary s's

Strümpell
    S's disease
    S's phenomenon
    S's reflex
    S's sign
    S.-Leichtenstern disease
    S.-Leichtenstern encephali-
      tis

Stryker frame

study
    nerve conduction s's

stun

stupor
    catatonic s.
    epileptic s.
    postconvulsive s.

stuporous

Sturge
    S.-Kalischer-Weber syn-
      drome
    S.-Weber syndrome

subarachnoid

subbrachial

subcalcarine

subconscious

subconsciousness

subcortex

subcortical

subcranial

subdelirium

subdural

subependymal

subependymoma

subfoliar

subfolium

subfrontal

subgrondation

subgyrus

subicular

subiculum *pl.* subicula
    s. cornu ammonis
    s. hippocampi

subliminal

subneural

subnucleus

subparalytic

subpial

subsplenial

substance
    arborescent white s. of
      cerebellum
    black s.
    central gelatinous s. of spi-
      nal cord
    chromophil s.
    cortical s. of cerebellum
    gelatinous s. of posterior
      horn of spinal cord
    gray s.
    gray s., central
    gray s. of spinal cord
    I s.
    intermediate s. of spinal
      cord, central
    intermediate s. of spinal
      cord, lateral
    medullary s.
    Nissl's s.
    s. P
    perforated s., anterior
    perforated s., interpedun-
      cular
    perforated s., posterior
    perforated s., rostral
    periaqueductal gray s.
    periventricular gray s.
    prelipid s.
    Reichert's s.
    reticular s.
    reticular s. of mesencepha-
      lon

substance *(continued)*
    Rolando's gelatinous s.
    second visceral s. of spinal
      cord
    tigroid s.
    transmitter s.
    white s.
    white s. of spinal cord
    white s. of cerebellum

substantia *pl.* substantiae
    s. alba
    s. alba medullae spinalis
    s. cinerea
    s. ferruginea
    s. gelatinosa cornu poster-
      ioris medullae spinalis
    s. gelatinosa centralis me-
      dullae spinalis
    s. gelatinosa Rolandi
    s. grisea
    s. grisea centralis
    s. grisea medullae spinalis
    s. grisea peri-aqueductalis
    s. innominata
    s. innominata of Reichert
    s. innominata of Reil
    s. intermedia centralis me-
      dullae spinalis
    s. intermedia lateralis me-
      dullae spinalis
    s. nigra
    s. perforata anterior
    s. perforata interpeduncu-
      laris
    s. perforata posterior
    s. perforata rostralis
    s. reticularis
    s. visceralis secundaria me-
      dullae spinalis

subsylvian

subtentorial

subtetanic

subthalamic

subthalamus

subwaking

sulcocommissural

sulcus *pl.* sulci
 anterolateral s. of medulla
  oblongata
 anterolateral s. of spinal
  cord
 s. anterolateralis medullae
  oblongatae
 s. anterolateralis medullae
  spinalis
 basilar s. of pons
 s. basilaris pontis
 bulbopontine s.
 s. bulbopontinus
 calcarine s.
 s. calcarinus
 callosal s.
 callosomarginal s.
 central cerebral s.
 s. centralis cerebri
 central s. of cerebrum
 central s. of insula
 s. centralis insulae
 cerebral sulci
 sulci cerebrales
 sulci cerebri
 sulci of cerebrum
 chiasmatic s.
 s. chiasmatis
 cingulate s.
 s. cingulatus
 s. cinguli
 s. of cingulum
 circular s. of insula
 s. circularis insulae
 collateral s.
 s. collateralis
 s. corporis callosi
 s. of corpus callosum
 dorsolateral s. of medulla
  oblongata
 dorsolateral s. of spinal
  cord
 s. dorsolateralis medullae
  oblongatae
 s. dorsolateralis medullae
  spinalis
 fimbriodentate s.

sulcus *(continued)*
 s. fimbriodentatus
 frontal s., inferior
 frontal s., superior
 s. frontalis inferior
 s. frontalis superior
 s. for greater petrosal
  nerve
 s. of habenula
 s. habenulae
 habenular s.
 s. habenularis
 hippocampal s.
 s. hippocampalis
 s. hippocampi
 horizontal s. of cerebellum
 hypothalamic s.
 s. hypothalamicus
 s. hypothalamicus [Mon-
  roi]
 sulci interlobares cerebri
 intermediate s. of spinal
  cord, dorsal
 intermediate s. of spinal
  cord, posterior
 s. intermedius dorsalis medullae spinalis
 s. intermedius posterior
  medullae spinalis
 interparietal s.
 intraparietal s.
 s. intraparietalis
 lateral cerebral s.
 lateral s. of cerebrum
 lateral s. of crus cerebri
 s. lateralis mesencephali
 lateral s. of medulla oblongata, anterior
 lateral s. of medulla oblongata, posterior
 lateral s. of mesencephalon
 lateral s. of spinal cord, anterior
 lateral s. of spinal cord,
  posterior
 s. lateralis cerebri
 s. lateralis pedunculi cerebri
 s. for lesser petrosal nerve

sulcus *(continued)*

s. limitans fossae rhomboideae

s. limitans of insula

lunate s.

s. lunatus

medial s. of crus cerebri

medial s. of mesencephalon

median s. of fourth ventricle

median s. of medulla oblongata, dorsal

median s. of medulla oblongata, posterior

median s. of spinal cord, dorsal

median s. of spinal cord, posterior

s. medianus dorsalis medullae oblongatae

s. medianus dorsalis medullae spinalis

s. medianus posterior medullae oblongatae

s. medianus posterior medullae spinalis

s. medianus ventriculi quarti

medullopontine s.

s. of Monro

s. nervi oculomotorii

s. nervi petrosi majoris

s. nervi petrosi minoris

occipital s., anterior

occipital sulci, lateral

occipital sulci, superior

occipital s., transverse

s. occipitalis anterior

sulci occipitales laterales

sulci occipitales superiores

s. occipitalis transversus

occipitotemporal s.

s. occipitotemporalis

oculomotor s.

s. oculomotorius

s. for oculomotor nerve

s. olfactorius lobi frontalis

olfactory s. of frontal lobe

sulcus *(continued)*

orbital sulci of frontal lobe

sulci orbitales lobi frontalis

parietooccipital s.

s. parietooccipitalis

parolfactory s., anterior

parolfactory s., posterior

polar s.

pontobulbar s.

pontopeduncular s.

postcentral s.

s. postcentralis

postclival s.

posterointermediate s. of spinal cord

posterolateral s. of medulla oblongata

posterolateral s. of spinal cord

s. posterolateralis medullae oblongatae

s. posterolateralis medullae spinalis

postnodular s.

postpyramidal s.

precentral s.

s. precentralis

prechiasmatic s.

s. prechiasmaticus

s. prechiasmatis

preclival s.

prepyramidal s.

prerolandic s.

Reil's s.

s. retroolivaris

rhinal s.

s. rhinalis

s. of spinal nerve

subparietal s.

s. subparietalis

suprasplenial s.

s. Sylvii

temporal s., inferior

temporal s., middle

temporal s., superior

temporal s., transverse

s. temporalis inferior

s. temporalis superior

s. temporalis transversus

sulcus *(continued)*
Turner's s.
s. valleculae
ventral s. of spinal cord
s. ventralis medullae spinalis
ventrolateral s. of medulla oblongata
ventrolateral s. of spinal cord
s. ventrolateralis medullae oblongatae
s. ventrolateralis medullae spinalis
vermicular s.
vertical s.

sumatriptan

summation
central s.

sundowning

supersensitivity
disuse s.

supracerebellar

supraliminal

supranuclear

suprapontine

suprasellar

suprasylvian

supratentorial

surface
tentorial s.

surgery
psychiatric s.
stereotactic s.
stereotaxic s.

suruçucu

suslik

suspenopsia

suture
nerve s.

sweating
gustatory s.

swelling
tympanic s.

Sydenham's chorea

sylvian
s. fissure
s. fossa

Sylvius
angle of S.
aqueduct of S.
cistern of fossa of S.
cisterna fossae Sylvii
fissure of S.
fossa of S.
iter of S.
sulcus Sylvii
ventricle of S.

symbolia

Symmetrel

sympathectomize

sympathectomy
chemical s.

sympathetectomy

sympathetic

sympatheticomimetic

sympatheticotonia

sympathetoblast

sympathic

sympathicectomy

sympathicoblast

sympathicoblastoma

sympathicogonioma

sympathicolysis

sympathicolytic

sympathicomimetic

sympathicopathy

sympathicotonia

sympathicotonic

sympathicotripsy

sympathicotrope

sympathicotropic

sympathoadrenal

sympathoblast

sympathoblastoma

sympathogonioma

sympatholytic

sympathomimetic

symptom
    Anton's s.
    Bonhoeffer's s.
    Brauch-Romberg s.
    dissociation s.
    Haenel s.
    negative s.
    precursory s.
    premonitory s.
    Remak's s.
    Roger's s.
    Séguin's signal s.
    signal s.

synalgia

synalgic

synapse
    axoaxonic s.
    axodendritic s.
    axodendrosomatic s.
    axosomatic s.
    chemical s.
    dendrodendritic s.
    electrical s.
    en passant s.
    loop s.

synapsis

synaptic

synaptology

synaptosome

synchiria

synchrony
    bilateral s.

syncinesis

synclonus

syncopal

syncope
    carotid sinus s.
    convulsive s.
    cough s.
    digital s.
    laryngeal s.
    stretching s.
    swallow s.
    tussive s.
    vasodepressor s.
    vasovagal s.

syncopic

syndrome
    abstinence s.
    acrocallosal s.
    Adie's s.
    Aicardi's s.
    Aicardi-Goutieres s.
    akinetic-rigid s.
    Alagille s.
    Alajouanine's s.
    Albright s.
    Alport's s.
    Andermann s.
    Andersen's s.
    Andrade's s.
    Angelman's s.
    angular gyrus s.
    anterior cord s.
    anterior cornual s.
    anterior interosseous s.
    anterior spinal artery s.
    Antley-Bixler s.
    Anton's s.
    Anton-Babinski s.
    Apert s.
    Arnold-Chiari s.

syndrome *(continued)*

    Arnold's nerve reflex
      cough s.
    ataxia-telangiectasia s.
    auriculotemporal s.
    autosomal recessive s. of
      progressive encephalopa-
      thy
    Avellis' s.
    Babinski-Nageotte s.
    Balint's s.
    Baller-Gerold s.
    Bannayan s.
    Bannwarth's s.
    Bardet-Biedl s.
    Barré-Guillain s.
    Barth s.
    Bartter s.
    basal cell nevus s.
    basilar artery s.
    Bassen-Kornzweig s.
    battered child s.
    Beckwith-Wiedemann s.
    Behr s.
    Benedikt's s.
    Berardinelli s.
    Bernard's s.
    Bernard-Horner s.
    Bing-Neel s.
    Bloom s.
    bobble-head doll s.
    body of Luys s.
    Bonnet-Dechaum-Blanc s.
    brachial s.
    Brissaud-Sicard s.
    Bristowe's s.
    Brown-Séquard's s.
    Brown-Vialetto-van Laere s.
    Brueghel's s.
    Bruns' s.
    Brushfield-Wyatt s.
    bulbar s.
    CACH s.
    CADASIL s.
    Canto-Rapin s.
    cardiofacial s.
    carotid sinus s.
    carpal tunnel s.
    Carpenter's s.

syndrome *(continued)*

    Carpenter-Philappart s.
    cauda equina s.
    caudal regression s.
    cavernous sinus s.
    Cayler s.
    central alveolar hypoventi-
      lation s.
    central cord s.
    central sleep apnea s.
    centroposterior s.
    cerebellar s.
    cerebellopontine angle s.
    cerebro-oculo-muscular s.
    cerebrofaciothoracic dys-
      plasia s.
    cerebrohepatorenal s.
    cervical s.
    cervical disk s.
    cervical rib s.
    cervicobrachial s.
    cervicomedullary s.
    Cestan's s.
    Cestan-Chenais s.
    Cestan-Raymond s.
    Charcot's s.
    Charcot-Marie s.
    Charcot-Weiss-Baker s.
    Charlin's s.
    Chédiak-Higashi s.
    Chiari-Arnold s.
    chiasma s.
    chiasmatic s.
    choreiform s.
    chronic fatigue s.
    Churg-Strauss s.
    Claude's s.
    closed head s.
    Cobb s.
    Cockayne s.
    Coffin-Siris s.
    Cogan's s.
    Collet's s.
    Collet-Sicard s.
    concussion s.
    congenital myasthenic s.
    congenital bilateral perisyl-
      vian s.

syndrome *(continued)*

 congenital central hypoventilation s.
 Constantinidis-Wisniewski s.
 continuous muscle activity s.
 continuous muscle fiber activity s.
 conus medullaris s.
 Cornelia de Lange's s.
 s. of corpus striatum
 costoclavicular s.
 Cotard's s.
 craniocerebello-cardiac s.
 CRASH s.
 CREST s.
 cri du chat s.
 s. of crocodile tears
 Crow-Fukase s.
 cubital tunnel s.
 Curschmann-Steinert s.
 Dandy-Walker s.
 Davidenko s.
 de Clérambault s.
 Dejean's s.
 Dejerine's s.
 Dejerine-Klumpke s.
 Dejerine-Roussy s.
 Dejerine-Thomas s.
 De Morsier s.
 Dennie-Marfan s.
 Denny-Brown's s.
 De Toni-Fanconi s.
 dialysis dysequilibrium s.
 diencephalic s.
 DiGeorge s.
 dilapidated speech s.
 disconnection s.
 Divry-Van Boegart s.
 Down s.
 Dubowitz s.
 Duchenne's s.
 Duchenne-Erb s.
 Dyke-Davidoff-Masson s.
 Dyken s.
 Dyken-Edathodu s.
 Dyken-Wisniewski s.
 Eaton-Lambert s.

syndrome *(continued)*

 Edward's s.
 Ekbom s.
 empty sella s.
 encephalotrigeminal vascular s.
 extrapyramidal s.
 familial restless legs s.
 Fanconi s.
 fatal infantile s.
 fetal alcohol s.
 Fisher s.
 floppy infant s.
 Foix s.
 Foix-Alajouanine s.
 Förster's s.
 Förster's atonic-astatic s.
 Foster Kennedy s.
 Foville's s.
 fragile X s.
 Fraser s.
 Frey's s.
 Friderichsen-Waterhouse s.
 Friedmann's vasomotor s.
 Fröhlich s.
 Froin's s.
 Fryns s.
 Fukuhara s.
 Fukuyama's s.
 Garcin's s.
 Gélineau's s.
 Gerstmann's s.
 Gerstmann-Sträussler s.
 Gerstmann-Sträussler-Scheinker s.
 Gilles de la Tourette's s.
 glioma-polyposis s.
 Goebel s.
 Goldberg-Shprintzen s.
 Goldenhar's s.
 Goldenhar-Gorlin s.
 Gowers' s.
 Greig s.
 Guillain-Barré s.
 Gunn's s.
 gustatory sweating s.
 Hakim's s.
 half base s.
 Hallervorden-Spatz s.

syndrome *(continued)*
    hand-shoulder s.
    happy puppet s.
    HARD s.
    Heidenhain's s.
    Heller's s.
    hemolytic-uremic s.
    hereditary ataxic s.
    Hick's s.
    Hoffman-Werdnig s.
    Holmes-Adie s.
    Homén's s.
    Horner's s.
    Horton's s.
    Horner-Bernard s.
    Hunt's s.
    Hunter s.
    Hunter-McAlpine s.
    Hurler s.
    Hutchison s.
    hyperabduction s.
    hyperventilation s.
    inferior s. of red nucleus
    Isaacs' s.
    Isaacs-Mertens s.
    Jackson's s.
    Jackson-Weiss s.
    Jacod's s.
    Jahnke's s.
    Janz s.
    jaw-winking s.
    Jefferson's s.
    Johanson-Blizzard s.
    Joubert's s.
    jugular foramen s.
    Kallmann s.
    Kearns-Sayre s.
    Kennedy's s.
    Kiloh-Nevin s.
    Klein-Levin s.
    Klippel-Feil s.
    Klippel-Trenaunay-Weber s.
    Klumpke-Dejerine s.
    Klüver-Bucy s.
    Koerber-Salus-Elschnig s.
    Kugelberg-Welander s.
    Lambert-Eaton s.
    Lambert-Eaton myasthenic s.

syndrome *(continued)*
    Landau-Kleffner s.
    Landry's s.
    Langer-Giedion s.
    lateral medullary s.
    Leigh s.
    Lemieux-Neemeh s.
    Lennox s.
    Lennox-Gastaut s.
    Lévy-Roussy s.
    Leyden-Möbius s.
    Lichtheim's s.
    lissencephaly s.
    locked-in s.
    loculation s.
    longitudinal cord s.
    Louis-Bar's s.
    low-affinity fast-channel s.
    Lowe s.
    lower radicular s.
    Lowry-MacLean s.
    Lyell's s.
    Mackenzie's s.
    Maffucci's s.
    Marcus Gunn's s.
    marfanoid craniosynostosis s.
    median cleft face s.
    Meige's s.
    MELAS s.
    Melkersson-Rosenthal s.
    Melnick-Fraser s.
    Meniere's s.
    Menkes' kinky-hair s.
    Meretoja's s.
    MERRF s.
    metameric s.
    midface hypoplasia s.
    Millard-Gubler s.
    Miller-Dieker s.
    Miller Fisher s.
    MNGIE s.
    Möbius' s.
    Monakow's s.
    Mondini s.
    Moore's s.
    Morvan's s.
    Mount's s.
    Mount-Reback s.

syndrome *(continued)*

- myasthenic s.
- myoclonic encephalopathy s.
- Naffziger's s.
- neck-tongue s.
- Negri-Jacod s.
- Nélaton's s.
- neonatal withdrawal s's
- nerve compression s.
- Neuhauser s.
- neurocutaneous s.
- neuroleptic malignant s.
- Norman-Roberts s.
- Norman-Wood s.
- Nothnagel's s.
- Nyssen-van Bogaert s.
- obstructive sleep apnea s.
- oculopharyngeal s.
- one-and-a-half s.
- opsoclonus-myoclonus s.
- orbital floor s.
- organic delusional s.
- orofaciodigital I s.
- Osler-Rendu-Weber s.
- Othello s.
- outlet s.
- overlap s. in polymyositis
- paleostriatal s.
- pallidal s.
- Pallister-Hall s.
- paratrigeminal s.
- Parkes Weber s.
- parkinsonian s.
- Parry-Romberg s.
- Patau's s.
- Pendred's s.
- PEP s.
- Pepper s.
- petrosphenoid s.
- Pfeiffer s.
- phonologic syntactic s.
- Pickwickian s.
- Pierre Robin s.
- POEMS s.
- POLIP s.
- pontine s.
- postconcussion s.
- postconcussional s.

syndrome *(continued)*

- postconcussive s.
- posterior column s.
- posterior cord s.
- posterior inferior cerebellar artery s.
- posterior spinal cord s.
- post–lumbar puncture s.
- postpolio s.
- post-traumatic s.
- post-traumatic brain s.
- Prader-Willi s.
- premotor s.
- pronator s.
- pronator teres s.
- pseudo-Zellweger s.
- Putnam-Dana s.
- radicular s.
- Raeder's s.
- Raeder's paratrigeminal s.
- Ramsay Hunt s.
- Raymond-Cestan s.
- restless legs s.
- s. of retroparotid space
- Rett s.
- Reye s.
- Reye-like s.
- Rieger s.
- rigid spine s.
- Riley-Day s.
- Ritscher-Schinzel s.
- Robert's s.
- rolandic vein s.
- Rosenberg-Chutorian s.
- Roth's (Rot's) s.
- Roth-Bernhardt (Rot-Bernhardt) s.
- Roussy-Dejerine s.
- Roussy-Lévy s.
- Rubenstein-Taybi s.
- rubrospinal cerebellar peduncle s.
- Rukavina's s.
- Saethre-Chotzen s.
- Sandifer s.
- Sanfilippo s.
- scalenus s.
- scalenus anterior s.
- scalenus anticus s.

syndrome *(continued)*
  scapuloperoneal s.
  Scheie s.
  Schinzel-Giedion s.
  Schirmer's s.
  Schmidt's s.
  Schwartz-Jampel s.
  second impact s.
  segmentary s.
  s. of sensory dissociation
    with brachial amyotrophy
  shaken-impact infant s.
  shoulder-hand s.
  Shprintzen-Goldberg s.
  Shy-Drager s.
  Sicard's s.
  Sjögren s.
  Sjögren-Larsson s.
  sleep apnea s.
  slow-channel s.
  Sluder's s.
  Smith-Lemli-Opitz s.
  Sneddon's s.
  Sotos s.
  split-brain s.
  spondyloarthropathy s.
  Steele-Richardson-Olszew-
    ski s.
  Stein-Leventhal s.
  Stevens-Johnson s.
  Stickler s.
  stiff-baby s.
  stiff-man s.
  stroke s.
  Sturge's s.
  Sturge-Kalischer-Weber s.
  Sturge-Weber s.
  subclavian steal s.
  Swaiman-Lyons s.
  sylvian s.
  sylvian aqueduct s.
  syringomyelic s.
  Tapia's s.
  tarsal tunnel s.
  tegmental s.
  tethered cord s.
  thalamic s.
  thalamic pain s.
  Thévenard's s.

syndrome *(continued)*
  thoracic outlet s.
  Tolosa-Hunt s.
  Tourette's s.
  trisomy 9 mosaic s.
  trisomy 18 s.
  trisomy 21 s.
  tuberous sclerosis s.
  Turcot's s.
  upper airway resistance s.
  vagoaccessory s.
  vagoaccessory-hypoglos-
    sal s.
  Vail's s.
  Van Allen's s.
  van Bogaert-Nyssen s.
  vascular s.
  Vernet's s.
  vertebrobasilar s.
  Villaret's s.
  Vogt's s.
  Walker-Warburg s.
  Wallenberg's s.
  Warburg's s.
  Waterhouse-Friderichsen s.
  Welander's s.
  Wernicke's s.
  Wernicke-Korsakoff s.
  West's s.
  whiplash shaken infant s.
  Wildervanck s.
  Williams s.
  Wisniewski s.
  withdrawal emergent s.
  withdrawal s's
  Wohlfart-Kugelberg-Welan-
    der s.
  Wolfram s.
  Wright's s.
  Wyburn-Mason's s.
  X-linked scapuloperoneal s.
  XXX s.
  XYY s.
  Zellweger s.
  Zinsser-Cole-Engman s.

synencephalocele

synergetic

synergia

synergic

synergism

synergistic

synergy

synesthesia
    s. algica

synesthesialgia

synkinesia

synostosis
    coronal s.
    metopic s.
    multiple s.
    sagittal s.
    single s.

synkinesis
    imitative s.
    spasmodic s.

synkinetic

synreflexia

syphilis
    cerebrospinal s.
    meningovascular s.
    parenchymatous s.
    spinal s.

syringobulbia

syringocele

syringocoele

syringoencephalia

syringoencephalomyelia

syringohydromyelia

syringomyelia
    post-traumatic s.
    traumatic s.

syringomyelus

systatic

system
    anterolateral s.

system *(continued)*
    arc guidance s.
    association s.
    auditory s.
    autonomic nervous s.
    brain cooling s.
    central nervous s.
    centrencephalic s.
    enteric nervous s.
    exteroceptive nervous s.
    extracorticospinal s.
    extralemniscal s.
    extrapyramidal s.
    hypophyseoportal s.
    hypophysioportal s.
    hypothalamic hypophysial
      portal s.
    hypothalamic-pituitary s.
    hypothalamic-pituitary por-
      tal s.
    hypothalamo-hypophysial
      portal s.
    interoceptive nervous s.
    involuntary nervous s.
    lemniscal s.
    limbic s.
    nervous s.
    parasympathetic nervous s.
    peripheral nervous s.
    periventricular s.
    pituitary portal s.
    proprioceptive nervous s.
    pyramidal s.
    reticular activating s. (RAS)
    somatic nervous s.
    stereotactic s.
    sympathetic nervous s.
    vegetative nervous s.
    vestibular s.
    visceral nervous s.
    visual s.

systema *pl.* systemata
    s. nervosum
    s. nervosum autonomicum
    s. nervosum centrale
    s. nervosum periphericum

T
 T fiber

tabes
 diabetic t.
 t. dorsalis
 t. ergotica
 Friedreich's t.
 t. spinalis

taboparalysis

taboparesis

tache
 t. cérébrale
 t. méningéale
 t. motrice
 t. spinale

tachyphagia

tacrine

tactile

taction

tactometer

tactor

tactual

taenia *pl.* taeniae
 taeniae acusticae
 t. choroidea
 t. fornicis
 t. of fourth ventricle
 medullary t. of thalamus
 t. pontis
 t. telae
 t. thalami
 t. of third ventricle
 t. ventriculi quarti

taeniola *pl.* taeniolae
 t. corporis callosi of Reil

tail
 t. of caudate nucleus
 t. of dentate gyrus

taipan

Talma's disease

tangentiality

tangle
 neurofibrillary t's

tanycyte

tap
 bloody t.
 front t.
 heel t.
 spinal t.

tapetum
 t. corporis callosi

Tapia's syndrome

tarbagan

Tarin
 fascia of T.
 T's fossa
 T's recess
 T's space

Tarinus' valve

Tarlov cyst

tastant

taste
 franklinic t.

tautomeral

tears
 crocodile t.

technique
 Brown-Roberts-Wells t.
 Leksell t.
 Riechert-Mundinger t.
 stereotactic t.
 Todd-Wells t.

tectospinal

tectum *pl.* tecta
 t. mesencephali
 t. mesencephalicum
 t. of mesencephalon
 t. of midbrain

tegmen *pl.* tegmina
  t. ventriculi quarti

tegmentum *pl.* tegmenta
  hypothalamic t.
  t. mesencephalicum
  t. mesencephali
  t. of mesencephalon
  t. of midbrain
  t. pontis
  t. rhombencephali
  t. of rhombencephalon
  subthalamic t.

Tegretol
  T. XR

teichopsia

tela *pl.* telae
  t. choroidea of fourth ventricle
  t. choroidea of lateral ventricle
  t. choroidea of third ventricle
  t. choroidea ventriculi lateralis
  t. choroidea ventriculi quarti
  t. choroidea ventriculi tertii

telalgia

teleceptive

teleceptor

teledendrite

teledendron

telencephalic

telencephalization

telencephalon

teleneurite

teleneuron

teleost

telereceptor

telocoele

telodendrion

telodendron

teloglia

teloreceptor

temporopontile

tenderness
  pencil t.
  rebound t.

tenoreceptor

TENS
  transcutaneous electrical nerve stimulation

Tensilon test

tentorial

tentorium *pl.* tentoria
  t. cerebelli
  t. of cerebellum
  t. of hypophysis

terebrant

terebrating

terebration

terminal
  nerve t's

terminatio *pl.* terminationes
  t. nervorum libera

test
  Adson's t.
  Ayer's t.
  Ayer-Tobey t.
  Babinski's t.
  Bárány's pointing t.
  Bekhterev's (Bechterew's) t.
  binaural distorted speech t's
  Crafts' t.
  Elsberg's t.
  femoral nerve stretch t.
  finger-to-finger t.
  finger-nose t.

test *(continued)*
    finger-to-nose t.
    Fournier t.
    Funkenstein t.
    heel-knee t.
    heel-knee-shin t.
    heel-tap t.
    Janet's t.
    Linder's t.
    Naffziger's t.
    neostigmine t.
    orientation t.
    pointing t.
    Proetz t.
    Prostigmine t.
    Queckenstedt's t.
    Rinne t.
    Romberg's t.
    sniff t.
    sphenopalatine t.
    station t.
    Tensilon t.
    Tobey-Ayer t.
    Wada's t.
    Weber t.

testing
    neuropsychological t.

tetanic

tetaniform

tetanigenous

tetanization

tetanize

tetanode

tetanoid

tetanometer

tetanus
    cephalic t.
    cerebral t.
    physiological t.

tetany
    duration t.
    gastric t.
    hyperventilation t.
    latent t.

tetany *(continued)*
    parathyroid t.
    parathyroprival t.

tetrad
    narcoleptic t.

tetraparesis

tetraplegia

thalamectomy

thalamencephalic

thalamencephalon

thalami *(plural of* thalamus)

thalamic

thalamocortical

thalamolenticular

thalamomammillary

thalamotegmental

thalamotomy
    anterior t.
    dorsomedial t.

thalamus *pl.* thalami
    dorsal t.
    t. dorsalis
    optic t.
    ventral t.
    t. ventralis

thalposis

thalpotic

Thane's method

theca *pl.* thecae
    t. medullare spinalis
    t. vertebralis

Theimich's lip sign

theory
    avalanche t.
    convergence-projection t.
    core conductor t.
    gate t.
    gate-control t.
    Golgi's t.

theory *(continued)*
  local circuit t.
  neuron t.
  thermostat t.

therapy
  abortive t.
  prophylactic t.

thermalgesia

thermalgia

thermanalgesia

thermanesthesia

thermesthesia

thermesthesiometer

thermhyperesthesia

thermhypesthesia

thermoalgesia

thermoanalgesia

thermoanesthesia

thermoceptor

thermocoagulation
  radiofrequency t.

thermoesthesia

thermoesthesiometer

thermoexcitory

thermohyperalgesia

thermohyperesthesia

thermohypesthesia

thermohypoesthesia

thermoreceptor

thermostat
  hypothalamic t.

thigh
  drivers' t.
  Heilbronner's t.

thigmesthesia

thinking
  concrete t.

Thomas' sign

Thomsen's disease

thought broadcasting

thought insertion

thought withdrawal

threshold
  absolute t.
  arousal t.
  t. of consciousness
  differential t.
  double point t.
  insular t.
  neuron t.
  relational t.
  resolution t.
  sensitivity t.
  stimulus t.
  swallowing t.

Throckmorton
  T's reflex
  T's sign

thrombophlebitis
  intracranial t.

thrombosinusitis

thrombosis
  atrophic t.
  cavernous sinus t.
  cerebral t.
  intracranial t.
  intracranial sinus t.
  marantic t.
  marasmic t.
  sinus t.

thrombus *pl.* thrombi
  marantic t.
  marasmic t.

TIA
  transient ischemic attack

tiagabine

tic
> convulsive t.
> diaphragmatic t.
> t. douloureux
> facial t.
> t. de Guinon
> habit t.
> local t.
> mimic t.
> saltatory t.
> t. de sommeil

tickling

Ticlid

ticlopidine

ticpolonga

tigroid

Tiedemann's nerve

tigrolysis

time
> Achilles tendon reflex t.
> conduction t.
> inertia t.
> reaction t.
> rise t.
> stimulus-response t.
> utilization t.

Timofeew's corpuscle

tingling
> distal t. on percussion

tiqueur

tissue
> epivaginal connective t.
> Kuhnt's intermediary t.
> nerve t.
> nervous t.

titillation

titubant

titubation

Tizanidine

TNS
> transcutaneous electrical
> nerve stimulation

Tobey-Ayer test

Todd
> T. bodies
> T's paralysis
> T.-Wells apparatus
> T.-Wells technique

toe
> Morton's t.

Tolosa-Hunt syndrome

tomentum

tomography
> computed t. (CT)
> positron emission t. (PET)
> single photon emission
> computed t. (SPECT)
> xenon-computed t. (XeCT)

tonaphasia

tone
> resting t.

tonic

tonic-clonic

tonicoclonic

tonoclonic

tonotopic

tonotopicity

tonsil
> t. of cerebellum

tonsilla *pl.* tonsillae
> t. cerebelli

tonus

Tooth
> T's atrophy
> T's disease

topagnosia

topagnosis

Topamax

topectomy

topesthesia

topiramate

topoanesthesia

topognosis

topothermesthesiometer

torcular
t. Herophili

Torkildsen
T's operation
T's shunt

torpent

torpid

torpidity

torpor

torticollis
intermittent t.
mental t.
neurogenic t.
paroxysmal t.
spasmodic t.

tortipelvis

touch

Tourette's syndrome

toxoplasmic
t. encephalitis
t. encephalomyelitis
t. meningoencephalitis

toxoplasmosis
cerebral t.

trachelism

trabecula *pl.* trabeculae
arachnoid trabeculae
trabeculae arachnoideae

trachelismus

tracking
visual t.

tract
anterolateral t's
ascending t.
Bekhterev's (Be-
chterew's) t.
Bruce's t.
bulbar t.
bulboreticulospinal t.
bulbothalamic t.
Burdach's t.
central t. of auditory nerve
cerebellorubral t.
cerebellorubrospinal t.
cerebellospinal t.
cerebellotegmental t's of
bulb
cerebellothalamic t.
comma t. of Schultze
corticobulbar t.
corticohypothalamic t.
corticomesencephalic t.
corticonuclear t.
corticopontine t.
corticorubral t.
corticospinal t., anterior
corticospinal t., crossed
corticospinal t., direct
corticospinal t., lateral
corticospinal t., ventral
corticospinal t. of medulla
oblongata
corticospinal t's of spinal
cord
corticotectal t., external
corticotectal t., internal
cuneocerebellar t.
Deiters' t.
dentatothalamic t.
descending t.
dorsolateral t.
extracorticospinal t.
extrapyramidal t.
fastigiobulbar t's
fiber t's of spinal cord
Flechsig's t.
frontopontine t.

tract *(continued)*

- geniculocalcarine t.
- geniculostriate t.
- Goll's t.
- Gowers' t.
- habenulointerpeduncular t.
- habenulopeduncular t.
- habenulothalamic t.
- Helweg's t.
- hypothalamicohypophysial t.
- hypothalamohypophysial t.
- intermediolateral t.
- internuncial t.
- intersegmental t. of spinal cord, anterior
- intersegmental t. of spinal cord, dorsal
- intersegmental t. of spinal cord, lateral
- intersegmental t. of spinal cord, posterior
- intersegmental t. of spinal cord, ventral
- interstitiospinal t.
- Lissauer's t.
- Löwenthal's t.
- mammillopeduncular t.
- mammillotegmental t.
- mammillothalamic t.
- Marchi's t.
- mesencephalic t. of trigeminal nerve
- Meynert's t.
- Monakow's t.
- motor t.
- nigrostriate t.
- occipitopontile t.
- occipitopontine t.
- olfactory t.
- olivocerebellar t.
- olivocochlear t.
- olivospinal t.
- optic t.
- paraventriculohypophysial t.
- parietopontine t.
- peduncular t., transverse
- pontoreticulospinal t.

tract *(continued)*

- posterolateral t.
- pyramidal t.
- pyramidal t., anterior
- pyramidal t., crossed
- pyramidal t., direct
- pyramidal t., lateral
- pyramidal t., ventral
- pyramidal t. of medulla oblongata
- pyramidal t's of spinal cord
- reticulospinal t.
- reticulospinal t., anterior
- reticulospinal t., lateral
- reticulospinal t., medial
- reticulospinal t., medullary
- reticulospinal t., ventral
- rubrobulbar t.
- rubroreticular t.
- rubrospinal t.
- Schultze's t.
- Schütz's t.
- semilunar t.
- sensory t.
- septomarginal t.
- solitary t. of medulla oblongata
- spinal t. of trigeminal nerve
- spinocerebellar t., anterior
- spinocerebellar t., direct
- spinocerebellar t., dorsal
- spinocerebellar t., posterior
- spinocerebellar t., ventral
- spinocervical t.
- spinocervicothalamic t.
- spinoolivary t.
- spinoreticular t.
- spinotectal t.
- spinothalamic t.
- spinothalamic t., anterior
- spinothalamic t., lateral
- spinothalamic t., ventral
- spinovestibular t.
- Spitzka's t.
- Spitzka-Lissauer t.
- strionigral t.
- sulcomarginal t.
- supraopticohypophysial t.

tract *(continued)*
    tectobulbar t.
    tectocerebellar t.
    tectospinal t.
    tegmental t.
    tegmental t., central
    tegmentospinal t.
    temporopontine t.
    testobulbar t.
    thalamo-olivary t.
    t. of Bruce and Muir
    t. of Philippe-Gombault
    t. of Vicq d'Azyr
    triangular t.
    triangular t. of Philippe-Gombault
    trigeminothalamic t.
    tuberohypophysial t.
    tuberoinfundibular t.
    ventral amygdalofugal t.
    vestibulocerebellar t.
    vestibulospinal t.
    vestibulospinal t., lateral
    vestibulospinal t., medial

tractotomy
    medullary t.
    mesencephalic t.
    stereotactic t.

tractus
    t. anterolaterales
    t. bulboreticulospinalis
    t. corticopontinus
    t. corticospinalis anterior
    t. corticospinalis lateralis
    t. corticospinalis ventralis
    t. dorsolateralis
    t. frontopontinus
    t. habenulo-interpeduncularis
    t. hypothalamohypophysialis
    t. interstitiospinalis
    t. mesencephalicus nervi trigeminalis
    t. mesencephalicus nervi trigemini
    t. olfactorius
    t. olivocerebellaris

tractus *(continued)*
    t. olivocochlearis
    t. opticus
    t. paraventriculohypophysialis
    t. pontoreticulospinalis
    t. posterolateralis
    t. pyramidalis
    t. pyramidalis anterior
    t. pyramidalis lateralis
    t. pyramidalis ventralis
    t. reticulospinalis anterior
    t. reticulospinalis anterior
    t. reticulospinalis ventralis
    t. rubrobulbaris
    t. rubrospinalis
    t. solitarius medullae oblongatae
    t. spinalis nervi trigeminalis
    t. spinalis nervi trigemini
    t. spinocerebellaris anterior
    t. spinocerebellaris dorsalis
    t. spinocerebellaris posterior
    t. spinocerebellaris ventralis
    t. spinocervicalis
    t. spino-olivaris
    t. spinoreticularis
    t. spinotectalis
    t. spinothalamicus
    t. spinothalamicus anterior
    t. spinothalamicus lateralis
    t. spinothalamicus ventralis
    t. supraopticohypophysialis
    t. tectobulbaris
    t. tectospinalis
    t. tegmentalis centralis
    t. trigeminothalamicus
    t. vestibulospinalis lateralis
    t. vestibulospinalis medialis

transantral

transbasal

transcallosal

transcalvarial

transcortical

transcranial

transducer
  neuroendocrine t.

transduction
  sensory t.

transdural

transethmoidal

transfrontal

transient
  t. ischemic attack (TIA)

transilient

transinsular

transisthmian

transmission
  duplex t.
  ephaptic t.
  neurochemical t.
  neurohumoral t.
  neuromuscular t.
  synaptic t.

transport
  anterograde t.
  fast axonal t.
  retrograde t.
  slow axonal t.

transsphenoidal

transtemporal

transthalamic

transventricular

treatment
  Hartel's t.
  Matas' t.
  Schlösser's t.

tree
  dendritic t.

tremogram

tremograph

tremor
  action t.
  coarse t.
  continuous t.
  enhanced physiologic t.
  essential t.
  familial t.
  fine t.
  flapping t.
  hereditary essential t.
  heredofamilial t.
  intention t.
  kinetic t.
  t. linguae
  orthostatic t.
  parkinsonian t.
  passive t.
  persistent t.
  physiologic t.
  pill-rolling t.
  postural t.
  rest t.
  resting t.
  senile t.
  static t.
  striocerebellar t.
  trombone t. of tongue
  volitional t.

tremorgram

tremulous

trepidant

trepidation

triad
  Charcot's t.
  Jacod's t.
  t. of Luciani

triangle
  Gombault-Philippe t.
  Reil's t.
  Wernicke's t.

trichesthesia

trichoesthesia

trichoesthesiometer

tricorn

trifacial

trigeminal

trigeminus

trigone
  cerebral t.
  collateral t. of fourth ventricle
  collateral t. of lateral ventricle
  t. of habenula
  habenular t.
  hypoglossal t.
  t. of hypoglossal nerve
  interpeduncular t.
  t. of lateral lemniscus
  olfactory t.
  pontocerebellar t.
  t. of Reil
  vagal t.
  t. of vagus nerve

trigonum *pl.* trigona
  t. collaterale ventriculi lateralis
  t. habenulae
  t. habenulare
  t. hypoglossale
  t. lemnisci lateralis
  t. nervi hypoglossi
  t. nervi vagi
  t. olfactorium
  t. pontocerebellare
  t. vagale

Trileptal

triplegia

triplet

tripoding

trismic

trismus

Triton tumor

trough
  synaptic t.

Trousseau
  T's phenomenon
  T's sign
  T's spot
  T's twitching

truncus *pl.* trunci
  t. corporis callosi
  t. encephali
  t. encephalicus
  t. inferior plexus brachialis
  t. lumbosacralis
  t. medius plexus brachialis
  t. nervi accessorii
  t. nervi spinalis
  trunci plexus brachialis
  t. superior plexus brachialis
  t. sympatheticus
  t. sympathicus
  t. vagalis anterior
  t. vagalis posterior

trunk
  t. of accessory nerve
  t's of brachial plexus
  t. of corpus callosum
  encephalic t.
  inferior t. of brachial plexus
  lower t. of brachial plexus
  lumbosacral t.
  middle t. of brachial plexus
  t. of spinal nerve
  superior t. of brachial plexus
  sympathetic t.
  upper t. of brachial plexus
  vagal t., anterior
  vagal t., posterior

tuber
  t. cinereum
  t. vermis

tubercle
  acoustic t.
  auditory t.
  Babès' t's
  cuneate t.

tubercle *(continued)*
    t. of cuneate nucleus
    gracile t.
    gray t.
    intercolumnar t.
    mammillary t. of hypothalamus
    Morgagni's t.
    t. of nucleus cuneatus
    t. of nucleus gracilis
    rabic t's
    t. of Rolando
    t. of sella turcica
    thalamic t., anterior
    thalamic t., posterior
    trigeminal t.

tuberculoma
    t. en plaque

tuberculosis
    cerebral t.

tuberculum *pl.* tubercula
    t. anterius thalami
    t. cinereum
    t. cuneatum
    t. gracile
    t. sellae turcicae
    t. trigeminale

tubulization

tumeur
    t. perlée

tumor
    acoustic nerve t.
    craniopharyngeal duct t.
    dumbbell t.
    epidermoid t.
    hourglass t.
    Lindau's t.

tumor *(continued)*
    margaroid t.
    nerve sheath t.
    neuroepithelial t.
    pearl t.
    pearly t.
    Pepper t.
    peripheral neuroectodermal t.
    primitive neuroectodermal t.
    primitive neuroepithelial t.
    Rathke's t.
    Rathke's pouch t.
    sand t.
    Schwann cell t.
    sheath t.
    Triton t.

tunicate

tunicin

Türck
    T's bundle
    T's column
    T's degeneration
    fasciculus of T.

Turcot's syndrome

Turner
    marginal gyrus of T.
    T's sulcus

Turyn's sign

twinge

twitching
    Trousseau's t.

type
    sympatheticotonic t.

U

ulcer
    neurogenic u.
    neurotrophic u.
    trophoneurotic u.

ulegyria

ultrasound
    cranial u.

uncal

unci (*plural of* uncus)

uncinal

uncinate

unconscious

uncotomy

uncus *pl.* unci
    u. gyri fornicati
    u. gyri hippocampi

uncus *(continued)*
    u. gyri parahippocampalis

underhorn

unguis
    u. ventriculi lateralis cere-
      bri

unirritable

unit
    motor u.

unmedullated

unmyelinated

Unverricht
    U's disease
    U.-Lundborg disease

uvula *pl.* uvula
    u. cerebelli
    u. of cerebellum
    u. vermis

vadum

vagal

vagectomy

vagi (*plural of* vagus)

vagina *pl.* vaginae
v. externa nervi optici
v. interna nervi optici
vaginae nervi optici

vagoaccessorius

vagoglossopharyngeal

vagogram

vagolysis

vagolytic

vagomimetic

vagosplanchnic

vagosympathetic

vagotomy
bilateral v.
highly selective v.
parietal cell v.
posterior truncal v.
selective v.
truncal v.

vagotonia

vagotonic

vagotony

vagotropic

vagovagal

vagus *pl.* vagi

Vail
V's neuralgia
V's syndrome

Valentin
V's corpuscles
V's pseudoganglion
tympanic ganglion of V.

Valium

vallecula *pl.* valleculae
v. cerebelli

valproic acid

value
liminal v.
threshold v.

valve
Tarinus' v.
v. of Vieussens
Willis' v.

vampire

Van Allen
V. A's syndrome
V. A. type familial amyloid
polyneuropathy

van Bogaert
v. B's encephalitis
v. B's sclerosing leukoencephalitis
v. B.-Nyssen syndrome

van der Kolk's law

Vanzetti's sign

variant
migraine v.
petit mal v.

variation
contingent negative v.

varolian

vasculitis
granulomatous v. of central
nervous system
granulomatous cerebral v.
isolated v. of central nervous system

vasodilative

vasodilator

vasoneuropathy

vasoneurosis

vasoparesis

vasoreflex

vasosensory

vasovagal

Vater
    V's corpuscle
    V.-Pacini corpuscle

vegetative

vein
    hypophyseoportal v's
    portal v's of hypophysis

velamentum *pl.* velamenta
    velamenta cerebri

vellus
    v. olivae

velocity
    nerve conduction v.

velum *pl.* vela
    v. interpositum cerebri
    v. medullare anterius
    v. medullare caudale
    v. medullare inferius
    v. medullare posterius
    v. medullare rostralis
    v. medullare superius
    medullary v., anterior
    medullary v., caudal
    medullary v., inferior
    medullary v., posterior
    medullary v., rostral
    medullary v., superior
    v. of Tarinus

vena *pl.* venae
    venae portales hypophy-
        siales

Venezuelan
    V. equine encephalitis
    V. equine encephalomyeli-
        tis

ventricle
    v. of Arantius
    v's of the brain

ventricle *(continued)*
    Duncan's v.
    fifth v.
    first v. of cerebrum
    fourth v. of cerebrum
    lateral v. of cerebrum
    pineal v.
    second v. of cerebrum
    sixth v.
    v. of Sylvius
    terminal v. of spinal cord
    third v. of cerebrum
    Verga's v.
    Vieussens' v.

ventriculitis

ventriculoatriostomy

ventriculocisternostomy

ventriculoencephalitis
    cytomegalovirus v.

ventriculomegaly

ventriculometry

ventriculopuncture

ventriculoscope

ventriculoscopy

ventriculostium

ventriculostomy

ventriculosubarachnoid

ventriculotomy

ventriculovenostomy

ventriculus *pl.* ventriculi
    v. dexter cerebri
    v. lateralis cerebri
    v. quartus cerebri
    v. sinister cerebri
    v. terminalis medullae spi-
        nalis
    v. tertius cerebri

ventrocaudal

verbigeration

Verga's ventricle

vermes

vermian

vermis
v. cerebelli

Vernet's syndrome

Verneuil's neuroma

Verocay bodies

vertebrate

vertiginous

vertigo
angiopathic v.
apoplectic v.
arteriosclerotic v.
benign paroxysmal v. of childhood
benign paroxysmal positional v.
benign positional v.
benign postural v.
central v.
cerebral v.
cervical v.
disabling positional v.
encephalic v.
endemic paralytic v.
epidemic v.
epileptic v.
essential v.
gastric v.
horizontal v.
laryngeal v.
lateral v.
mechanical v.
nocturnal v.
objective v.
ocular v.
organic v.
paralytic v.
paralyzing v.
paroxysmal v.
peripheral v.
positional v.
posttraumatic v.
postural v.

vertigo *(continued)*
primary v.
residual v.
rotary v.
rotatory v.
stomachal v.
v. ab stomacho laeso
subjective v.
systematic v.
tenebric v.
toxic v.
vertical v.
vestibular v.

vesicle
olfactory v.
synaptic v's

vesikin

vestibulocerebellum

vestibulo-ocular

Vicq d'Azyr
V. d'A's band
fasciculus of V. d'A.
foramen of V. d'A.
foramen caecum of V. d'A.
V. d'A's stripe
tract of V. d'A.

Vienna encephalitis

Vieussens
V's annulus
ansa of V.
loop of V.
valve of V.
V's ventricle

Villaret's syndrome

villus *pl.* villi
arachnoid villi
villi of choroid plexus

vinculum *pl.* vincula
vincula lingulae cerebelli

Virchow
V's granulations
V.-Robin spaces

viscerimotor

visceromotor

viscerosensory

viscerotome

vision
  facial v.

visuoauditory

visuomotor

visuopsychic

viviparity

viviparous

vivipation

VLA-4 adhesion

VNS
  vagus nerve stimulator

Vogt
  V.'s point

Vogt *(continued)*
  V's syndrome
  V.-Hueter point

Voit's nucleus

vole
  bank v.
  field v.

volley
  antidromic v.

voluntomotory

vomiting
  cerebral v.

von Economo
  von E's disease
  von E's encephalitis

von Hippel-Lindau disease

von Monakow's fibers

von Recklinghausen's disease

Vulpian's atrophy

Wada's test

wakefulness

Walker
    W's lissencephaly
    W.-Warburg syndrome

walking
    heel w.

Wallenberg's syndrome

Warburg's syndrome

Wartenberg
    W's disease
    W's sign

Waterhouse-Friderichsen syndrome

watershed

wave
    A w.
    alpha w's
    axon w.
    beta w's
    brain w's
    delta w's
    E w.
    electroencephalographic w's
    expectancy w.
    F w's
    H w.
    lambda w's
    M w.
    positive sharp w.
    R_1 w.
    R_2 w.
    random w's
    sharp w.
    theta w's

web
    subsynaptic w.

Weber
    W's disease
    W. test

Wedensky
    W. facilitation
    W. inhibition
    W's phenomenon

Welander's syndrome

Werdnig
    W.-Hoffmann spinal muscular atrophy
    W.-Hoffmann disease

Wernicke
    W's aphasia
    W's area
    W's disease
    W's field
    W's second motor speech area
    W's syndrome
    W's triangle
    W's zone
    W.-Korsakoff syndrome
    W.-Mann hemiplegia

West's syndrome

West Nile encephalitis

Weston Hurst
    acute hemorrhagic leukoencephalitis of W. H.
    W. H. disease

Westphal
    W's nuclei
    W's phenomenon
    W's sign
    W's zone

whiplash

white matter degeneration

Whytt's disease

Wildervanck syndrome

Williams syndrome

Willis
    arterial circle of W.
    W's cords
    W's valve

Wilson's disease

wing
    w. of central lobule

winking
    jaw w.

Wisniewski syndrome

Wohlfart-Kugelberg-Welander
    syndrome

Wolfram syndrome

word salad

Wright's syndrome

Wrisberg's nerve

wristdrop

Wyburn-Mason's syndrome

xanchromatic

xanthochromatic

xanthochromic

XeCT
    xenon-computed tomogra-
      phy

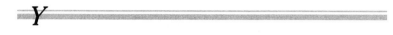

Y

yttrium
  y. 90

Zarontin

zeitgeber

Zellweger
   pseudo-Z. syndrome
   Z. syndrome

zero
   physiologic z.

Ziehen-Oppenheim disease

Ziemssen's motor point

Zimmerlin's atrophy

Zinsser-Cole-Engman syndrome

Zomig

zona *pl.* zonae
   z. incerta
   z. ophthalmica
   z. rolandica

zone
   active z.
   anelectrotonic z.
   chemoreceptor trigger z.
   cornuradicular z.
   dolorogenic z.
   entry z.
   epileptogenic z.
   Flechsig's primordial z's

zone *(continued)*
   hyperesthetic z.
   intermediate z. of spinal
      cord
   language z.
   lateral z. of hypothalamus
   Lissauer's marginal z.
   medial z. of hypothalamus
   motor z.
   z. of partial preservation
   peripolar z.
   periventricular z.
   polar z.
   Rolando's z.
   root z.
   trigger z.
   Wernicke's z.
   Westphal's z.

zonisamide

zonesthesia

zoogonous

zoogony

zoster
   ophthalmic z.

Zuckerkandl's convolution

zygomycosis
   rhinocerebral z.

zygon

Drugs Used in Neurology

Below are the names of generic and ℞ brand name drugs used in neurology, as shown in the *Saunders Pharmaceutical Xref Book*. The drugs are categorized by their "indications"—also called "designated use," "approved use," or "therapeutic action"—which group together drugs used for a similar purpose. The indications shown below are broad categories of therapeutic action. Individual drugs may be placed in subcategories or have specifically targeted diseases beyond the scope of this listing. For complete information about the drugs listed below, including each drug's availability, specific indications, forms of administration, and dosages, please consult the current edition of *Saunders Pharmaceutical Word Book*.

Analgesics
Analgesics, Antimigraine
Amaphen
Amaphen with Codeine #3
Amerge
Anoquan
Arcet
Axocet
Axotal
Betachron E-R
Bucet
Bupap
butalbital
Butalbital Compound
Cafatine
Cafatine-PB
Cafergot
Cafetrate
D.H.E. 45
dihydroergotamine mesylate
Endolor
Ercaf
Ergomar
Ergostat
ergotamine tartrate
Esgic
Esgic-Plus
Femcet
feverfew (*Chrysanthemum parthenium; Leucanthemum parthenium; Pyrethrum parthenium; Tanacetum parthenium*)

Analgesics, Antimigraine (cont.)
Fiorgen PF
Fioricet
Fioricet with Codeine
Fiorinal
Fiorinal with Codeine
Fiorpap
Fiortal
frovatriptan succinate
Imitrex
Inderal
Inderal LA
Ipran
Isocet
Isocom
Isollyl Improved
isometheptene mucate
Isopap
Lanorinal
Margesic
Marnal
Marten-Tab
Maxalt
Maxalt-MLT
Medigesic
methysergide maleate
Midchlor
Midrin
Migranal
Migratine
Miguard
naratriptan HCl

Analgesics, Antimigraine (cont.)
Phrenilin
Phrenilin Forte
Prominol
propranolol HCl
Repan
Repan CF
rizatriptan benzoate
Sansert
Sedapap
sumatriptan succinate
Tencet
Tencon
Triad
Triaprin
Two-Dyne
Wigraine
zolmitriptan
Zomig

Analgesics, Narcotic
Aceta with Codeine
Actiq
AERx
Alfenta
alfentanil HCl
Alor 5/500
Amacodone
Amaphen with Codeine #3
Anexsia 5/500; Anexsia 7.5/650; Anexsia 10/660
Aspirin with Codeine No. 2, No. 3, and No. 4
Astramorph PF
Azdone
B & O Supprettes No. 15A; B & O Supprettes No. 16A
Bancap HC
Buprenex
buprenorphine HCl
butorphanol tartrate
Capital with Codeine
Ceta Plus
Co-Gesic
codeine phosphate
Dalgan
Damason-P
Darvocet-N 50; Darvocet-N 100
Darvon
Darvon Compound-65
Darvon-N

Analgesics, Narcotic (cont.)
Demerol HCl
DepoMorphine
dezocine
DHC Plus
dihydrocodeine bitartrate
Dilaudid
Dilaudid Cough
Dilaudid-HP
Dirame
Dolacet
Dolene
Dolfen
Dolophine HCl
Duocet
Duragesic-25; Duragesic-50; Duragesic-75; Duragesic-100
Duramorph
E-Lor
Empirin with Codeine No. 3 & No. 4
fentanyl
fentanyl citrate
Fentanyl Oralet
Fioricet with Codeine
Fiorinal with Codeine
Genagesic
Hy-Phen
Hydrocet
hydrocodone bitartrate
Hydrogesic
hydromorphone HCl
HydroStat IR
Infumorph
Innovar
Kadian
Levo-Dromoran
levomethadyl acetate
levorphanol tartrate
Lorcet
Lorcet-HD
Lorcet Plus; Lorcet 10/650
Lortab
Lortab 2.5/500; Lortab 5/500; Lortab 7.5/500; Lortab 10/500
Lortab ASA
Margesic H
Margesic No. 3
Medipain 5
Mepergan
Mepergan Fortis

Analgesics, Narcotic (cont.)
  meperidine HCl
  methadone HCl
  Methadose
  MorphiDex
  morphine HCl
  morphine sulfate (MS)
  MS Contin
  MS/L; MS/L Concentrate
  MS/S
  MSIR
  nalbuphine HCl
  Norcet
  Norco
  Nubain
  Numorphan
  OMS Concentrate
  opium
  Oramorph SR
  Orlaam
  oxycodone HCl
  oxycodone terephthalate
  OxyContin
  OxyFast
  OxyIR
  oxymorphone HCl
  Panacet 5/500
  Panasal 5/500
  Papadeine #3
  paregoric (PG)
  pentazocine HCl
  pentazocine lactate
  Percocet
  Percodan; Percodan-Demi
  Percolone
  Phenaphen-650 with Codeine
  Phenaphen with Codeine No. 3 &
    No. 4
  Propacet 100
  propiram fumarate
  propoxyphene HCl
  propoxyphene napsylate
  Proxy 65
  Rid-A-Pain with Codeine
  RMS
  Roxanol
  Roxanol; Roxanol 100; Roxanol
    Rescudose; Roxanol T; Roxanol
    UD
  Roxicet

Analgesics, Narcotic (cont.)
  Roxicet 5/500
  Roxicodone
  Roxilox
  Roxiprin
  Soma Compound with Codeine
  Stadol
  Stadol NS
  Stagesic
  Sublimaze
  Sufenta
  sufentanil citrate
  Synalgos-DC
  T-Gesic
  Talacen
  Talwin
  Talwin Compound
  Talwin NX
  Tylenol with Codeine
  Tylenol with Codeine No. 2, No. 3,
    and No. 4
  Tylox
  UltraJect
  Vicodin; Vicodin ES; Vicodin HP
  Vicoprofen
  Wygesic
  Zydone
Analgesics, Neuralgia
  Atretol
  carbamazepine
  Carbatrol
  Depitol
  Epitol
  Tegretol
Analgesics, Nonsteroidal (NSAIDs)
  acetaminophen
  Aclophen
  Alumadrine
  Amaphen
  Amigesic
  aminobenzoate potassium
  Anaprox; Anaprox DS
  Anatuss
  Anoquan
  Ansaid
  Apo-Etodolac ⊛
  Arcet
  Argesic-SA
  Arthropan
  Arthrotec

**Analgesics, Nonsteroidal (NSAIDs)
(cont.)**

aspirin
aspirin, buffered
Axocet
Axotal
Brexidol
bromfenac sodium
Bucet
Bupap
Butalbital Compound
carprofen
Cataflam
Celebrex
celecoxib
choline magnesium trisalicylate
    (choline salicylate + magnesium
    salicylate)
choline salicylate
Clinoril
Daypro
diclofenac potassium
diclofenac sodium
Diclotec ⒸⒶⓃ
diflunisal
Disalcid
Dolobid
Duract
Easprin
EC-Naprosyn
Enable
Endolor
Epromate
Equagesic
Equazine M
Esgic
Esgic-Plus
etodolac
Feldene
Femcet
fenoprofen calcium
Fexicam ⒸⒶⓃ
Fiorgen PF
Fioricet
Fiorinal
Fiorpap
Fiortal
Flexaphen
flurbiprofen
Hyanalgese-D

**Analgesics, Nonsteroidal (NSAIDs)
(cont.)**

Hycomine Compound
Ibu
Ibu-Tab
ibuprofen
Ibuprohm
Indochron E-R
Indocin
Indocin SR
indomethacin
Isocet
Isocom
Isollyl Improved
Isopap
isoxicam
ketoprofen
ketorolac tromethamine
Lanorinal
Lobac
Lodine
Lodine XL
Magan
magnesium salicylate
Magsal
Margesic
Marnal
Marten-Tab
Marthritic
Maxicam
meclofenamate sodium
Meclomen
Medigesic
mefenamic acid
meloxicam
Meprogesic Q
Micrainin
Midchlor
Midrin
Migratine
Mobic
Mobidin
Mono-Gesic
Motrin
Mus-Lax
Myapap
nabumetone
Nalfon
Naprelan
Napron X

Analgesics, Nonsteroidal (NSAIDs) (cont.)
Naprosyn
naproxen
naproxen sodium
Norel Plus
Norgesic; Norgesic Forte
Orphengesic; Orphengesic Forte
Orudis
Oruvail
oxaprozin
Pabalate-SF
Pennsaid
Phenate
Phrenilin
Phrenilin Forte
piroxicam
piroxicam betadex
Ponstel
Prominol
Relafen
Repan
Repan CF
Rexolate
Rid-A-Pain with Codeine
Rimadyl
Robaxisal
rofecoxib
Rufen
Saleto-400; Saleto-600; Saleto-800
salicylamide
Salprofen
salsalate
Salsitab
Sedapap
sodium salicylate (SS)
sodium thiosalicylate
Sodol Compound
Soma Compound
Soma Compound with Codeine
sulindac
Tencet
Tencon
tenidap
Tolectin 200; Tolectin 600
Tolectin DS
tolmetin sodium
Toradol
Triad
Triaprin

Analgesics, Nonsteroidal (NSAIDs) (cont.)
Tricosal
Trilisate
Tussanil DH
Tussirex
Two-Dyne
Vioxx
Voltaren
Voltaren ⓒ
Voltaren Rapide ⓒ
Voltaren SR ⓒ
Voltaren XR
ZORprin

Analgesics, Topical
capsaicin
diclofenac potassium
menthol
Pennsaid
Solarase

Analgesics, Other
CereCRIB
clonidine
Duraclon
Levoprome
Metastron
methotrimeprazine
Oralease
Quadramet
samarium Sm 153 lexidronam
strontium chloride Sr 89
tramadol HCl
Ultram

Anticonvulsants
acetazolamide
acetazolamide sodium
Ativan
Atretol
Bellatal
carbamazepine
Carbatrol
Celontin
Cerebyx
clonazepam
Depacon
Depakene
Depakote
Depitol

Anticonvulsants (cont.)
  Deproic ⓒ
  Diamox
  Diastat
  Diazemuls ⓒ
  diazepam
  Dilantin
  Dilantin-30 Pediatric
  Dilantin with Phenobarbital
  Dilantin-125
  Diphenylan Sodium
  divalproex sodium
  Dizac
  Epiject ⓒ
  Epitol
  Epival ⓒ
  ethosuximide
  ethotoin
  felbamate
  Felbatol
  fosphenytoin sodium
  gabapentin
  Gabitril
  Klonopin
  Lamictal
  lamotrigine
  levetiracetam
  lorazepam
  Luminal Sodium
  magnesium sulfate
  Mebaral
  mephenytoin
  mephobarbital
  Mesantoin
  methsuximide
  Milontin
  Mogadon
  Mysoline
  neural gabaergic cells (or precur-
    sors), porcine fetal
  NeuroCell-HD
  Neurontin
  nitrazepam
  oxcarbazepine
  Paral
  paraldehyde
  Peganone
  phenacemide
  phenobarbital
  phenobarbital sodium

Anticonvulsants (cont.)
  phensuximide
  Phenurone
  phenytoin
  phenytoin sodium
  primidone
  Sabril
  Solfoton
  Tegretol
  Tegretol-XR
  tiagabine HCl
  Topamax
  topiramate
  Tridione
  Trileptal
  trimethadione
  Valium
  Valium Roche Oral ⓒ
  valproate sodium
  valproic acid
  Valrelease
  vigabatrin
  Zarontin
  Zetran
  Zonegran
  zonisamide

Antiparkinsonian Agents
**Antiparkinsonian Agents, Anticho-
  linergic Agents**
  Akineton
  Artane
  belladonna extract
  Bellafoline
  benztropine mesylate
  biperiden HCl
  biperiden lactate
  Cogentin
  Disipal ⓒ
  ethopropazine HCl
  Kemadrin
  orphenadrine HCl
  Parsidol
  procyclidine HCl
  Trihexy-2; Trihexy-5
  trihexyphenidyl HCl
**Antiparkinsonian Agents, Dopa-
  minergic Agents**
  amantadine HCl

**Antiparkinsonian Agents, Dopa-
minergic Agents (cont.)**
 bromocriptine mesylate
 cabergoline
 Carbex
 Dopar
 Dostinex
 Eldepryl
 Larodopa
 levodopa
 Mirapex
 N-Graft
 neural dopaminergic cells (or pre-
   cursors), porcine fetal
 NeuroCell-PD
 Parlodel
 pergolide mesylate
 Permax
 pramipexole dihydrochloride
 Requip
 ropinirole HCl
 selegiline HCl
 Sertoli cells, porcine
 Sinemet 10/100; Sinemet 25/100;
   Sinemet 25/250
 Sinemet CR
 Symadine
 Symmetrel
Antiparkinsonian Agents, Other
 Altropane
 Apokinon
 apomorphine HCl
 carbidopa
 Comtan
 entacapone
 iodine I 123 murine MAb to alpha-
   fetoprotein (AFP)
 Lodosyn
 Rilutek
 riluzole
 Tasmar
 tolcapone
 Zydis

Central Nervous System Stimulants
 Adderall
 Alertec 🇨🇦

**Central Nervous System
Stimulants (cont.)**
 amphetamine aspartate
 amphetamine sulfate
 caffeine
 caffeine, citrated
 Cylert
 d-methylphenidate HCl (d-MPH)
 Desoxyn
 Dexedrine
 dextroamphetamine saccharate
 dextroamphetamine sulfate
 Dextrostat
 Dopram
 doxapram HCl
 methamphetamine HCl
 Methylin
 methylphenidate
 methylphenidate HCl (MPH)
 modafinil
 Neocaf
 Oxydess II
 pemoline
 Provigil
 Ritalin
 Ritalin-SR
 Spancap No. 1

Multiple Sclerosis Agents
 Antegren
 bovine myelin
 Myloral

Muscle Relaxants
Muscle Relaxants, Skeletal
 Anectine
 Arduan
 atracurium besylate
 baclofen (L-baclofen)
 Banflex
 carisoprodol
 chlorphenesin carbamate
 chlorzoxazone
 cisatracurium besylate
 cyclobenzaprine HCl
 Dantrium
 dantrolene sodium

Muscle Relaxants, Skeletal (cont.)

Diazemuls 🇨🇦
diazepam
Dizac
doxacurium chloride
Flaxedil
Flexaphen
Flexeril
Flexoject
Flexon
gallamine triethiodide
Lioresal
Maolate
metaxalone
methocarbamol
metocurine iodide
Metubine Iodide
Mivacron
mivacurium chloride
Mus-Lax
Myolin
Nimbex
Norcuron
Norflex
Norgesic; Norgesic Forte
Nuromax
orphenadrine citrate
Orphengesic; Orphengesic Forte
pancuronium bromide
Paraflex
Parafon Forte DSC
Pavulon
pipecuronium bromide
Quelicin
Remular-S
Robaxin
Robaxisal
rocuronium bromide
Skelaxin
Sodol
Sodol Compound
Soma
Soma Compound
Soma Compound with Codeine
succinylcholine chloride
Sucostrin
Tracrium
tubocurarine chloride
Valium

Muscle Relaxants, Skeletal (cont.)

Valium Roche Oral 🇨🇦
Valrelease
vecuronium bromide
Zemuron
Zetran

Muscle Relaxants, Smooth

Cerespan
Cyclan
cyclandelate
Cyclospasmol
Cyclospasmol 🇨🇦
flavoxate HCl
Genabid
papaverine HCl
Pavabid
Pavabid HP
Pavagen TD
Pavarine
Pavased
Pavatine
Paverolan
Urispas

Muscle Stimulants

ambenonium chloride
carbachol
edrophonium chloride
Enlon
Enlon Plus
guanidine HCl
IGF-BP3 complex
Mestinon
Mytelase
neostigmine bromide
neostigmine methylsulfate
Prostigmin
pyridostigmine bromide
Regonol
Reversol
SomatoKine
Tensilon

Weight Reduction Agents
Weight Reduction Agents, CNS Modifiers

[see also: *Central Nervous System Stimulants*]

Adipex-P
Adipost
Anorex
benzphetamine HCl
Bontril
Bontril PDM
dexfenfluramine HCl
Didrex
diethylpropion
diethylpropion HCl
Dital
Dyrexan-OD
Fastin
fenfluramine HCl
Ionamin
Mazanor
mazindol
Melfiat-105
Meridia
Obalan
Obenix
Obephen
Oby-Cap
phendimetrazine tartrate
phentermine HCl
Phentrol
Phentrol 2; Phentrol 4; Phentrol 5
Plegine
Pondimin
Prelu-2
Redux
Rexigen Forte
Sanorex
sibutramine HCl
Tenuate
Tepanil
Trimstat
Wehless
Weightrol
Zantryl